THE IRRITABLE BOWEL SYNDROME SOLUTION

Dr. Stephen Wangen
Founder, IBS Treatment Center

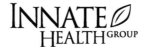

INNATE HEALTH GROUP

Innate Health Publishing
PO Box 27786, Seattle, WA, 98165-2786

First Printing: January 2006

10 9 8 7 6 5 4

Library of Congress Cataloging-in-Publication Data
Wangen, Stephen
The Irritable Bowel Syndrome Solution / Stephen Wangen
ISBN 978-0-9768537-8-7
1. Irritable colon – Popular works. 2. Irritable colon – Alternative
treatment – Popular works. 3. Health

PCN 2005926189

Cover and interior design www.KarenRoss.com

DISCLAIMER

This book is not intended as a substitute for the medical recommendations of physicians or other health care providers. It is intended to offer information to help the reader cooperate with physicians and health professionals so that they may work together to find better health.

The publisher and the author are not responsible for any products or services offered or referred to in this book and expressly disclaim all liability in connection with the use of any such products or services and for any damage, loss, or expense to person or property arising out of or relating to them.

All stories contained in this book are based on actual case studies, but the names and other details have been changed.

DEDICATION

This book is dedicated to all people suffering from digestive problems who are seeking an answer but have yet to find one. And to my patients, who have taught me most of what I know and given me the courage to share it with others.

The Irritable Bowel Syndrome Solution

ACKNOWLEDGEMENTS

I'd like to thank Kim Pearson for guiding me through the development of this book and making it a reality, Susan Fitzgerald for perfecting it, and Karen Ross for making it presentable. I'd also like to thank the following people for their academic and practical inspiration: Alan Gaby, M.D., for teaching me about the importance of food allergies in health; Nigel Plummer, PhD, for his wealth of information on the digestive tract and immune function; Kimberly Mathai, MS, RD, for her clinical and academic support; and Raymond and Margaret Suen for creating a reliable institution that helped me develop my treatment skills. Thanks also to Bill Slater for convincing me that I should write a book, Louise Shadduck for setting the example, Dan Poynter for showing me how to publish it, and Cynthia Kupper, RD, RN, and the members of the Gluten Intolerant Group for giving me the opportunity to speak and develop my message.

I'd also like to thank my classmates at Bastyr University, who helped me to become the physician I am today, and my patients for trusting me to help them and for teaching me how to be a better physician.

And of course my wife, Tara, without whom I may have never gotten to the point in life where I could write a book.

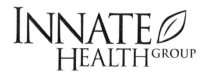

How to Contact the IBS Treatment Center

Phone: 206-264-1111
Toll free: 1-888-546-6283,
1-888-5INNATE

Website: www.ibstreatmentcenter.com

CONTENTS

INTRODUCTION

With apologies to other authors, I never read introductions, so it took a while before I could be convinced to write one. I want to know what the author has to say in the book, not what the author has to say in the introduction. I figure that if it's not in the book, then it probably isn't that important. Also, I've never been too interested in the author's motivation for writing the book. I'm more of a "just the facts" kind of guy. I want to know what's in it for me, not what was in it for the author. I won't be insulted if you decide to just skip ahead to the real meat of this book, but I have tried to make this introduction worth reading.

That's the approach that I've taken in this book — "what's in it for you." I've tried to describe, as simply as possible, the information that you need to know in order to solve your irritated digestive system. Because some issues are fairly complex, you'll have to apply a little mental energy. But I've learned over the years that when I don't understand something it is almost always due to one of three things — either the author hasn't done a very good job of communicating the issue (which is all too common, especially in textbooks), I am not properly focused on the issue at hand, or the concept is so bogus that there really isn't anything worth understanding.

Sometimes it's difficult to determine which issue is getting in the way of the learning process. I've made my best attempt to solve the first problem, and I can assure you that the latter issue has also been addressed. I think that you'll be amazed at how logical the answers actually are to most digestive problems. And you'll be left wondering why you haven't been told this before. That is a question that I hope you'll continue to ask yourself.

People are unique, and medical problems that appear to be similar can have a variety of causes. We're far too complex for one problem to always have the same cause. Our bodies are innately designed to function at an optimum level if we remove the obstacles to good health and provide the requirements necessary for good health. Unfortunately we don't often get quality medical advice that addresses this fact. Our health care system functions on a different principle — if you have a chronic health problem then generally it's either your own fault, you need a drug, or there is nothing that can be done (since we don't have a drug for it yet).

I don't know everything, but I have treated hundreds of patients with irritable bowel syndrome and the symptoms of diarrhea, constipation, gas, and chronic abdominal pain, and I've found that, with proper testing, these problems are almost always solvable. Therefore I created the IBS Treatment Center, the first clinic of its kind, and I've written this book.

I hope that this book can help you. At the very least it will give you some insight into how your body works. Read it from end to end or use the table of contents and jump to the parts you find most interesting. Either way it will be worth reading, even if you didn't read this introduction.

PART ONE

The IBS Challenge

Bad digestion is the root of all evil.
Hippocrates,
Greek physician (c.460 – 377c. B.C.)

CHAPTER ONE

It's Not a Laughing Matter

A woman went to her doctor to find out how to get rid of her constipation. "I feel awful," she said. "I haven't had a bowel movement in almost a week."

"I see," said the doctor. "Have you tried to do anything about it?"

"Of course," she said. "I sit in the bathroom for a half hour in the morning and another half hour at night."

"I meant do you take anything for it?" said the doctor.

"Well, of course," she said. "I take a book."

* * * * * * * * *

Did you know that diarrhea is hereditary?

Yeah, it runs in the jeans.

* * * * * * * * *

Doctor:"What seems to be the problem?"

Patient:"Well, I fart all the time."

Doctor:"Hmm ..."

Patient:"My farts do not stink and you can't hear them. It's just that I fart all the time. Look, we've been talking here for about 10 minutes and I've farted five times. You didn't hear them and you don't smell them, do you?"

Doctor:"Hmm ..." He picks up his pad and writes out a prescription.

Patient: "Will this medication clear up my farts?"

Doctor: "No. The prescription is to clear your sinuses. Next week I want you back here for a hearing test."

*   *   *   *   *   *   *   *   *

We think bodily functions, especially those having to do with our digestive tracts, are funny. A simple Google search on the Internet for "bathroom humor" will reward you with plenty of websites offering jokes, humorous articles, and hilarious phrases describing the many different kinds of eliminatory situations, appearances, noises, and smells that are part of the human condition. You will probably laugh at most of them. Because bathroom humor is funny, right?

Not always. Not if you're the butt of the joke.

Jennifer

"Jennifer" was nearly 17 and a junior in high school. She wore her dark brown hair fashionably long, framing an expressive face, with its deep brown eyes and impish smile. She laughed a lot, and was known around school for her sense of humor.

No one would guess the pain and embarrassment she endured nearly every day. And she sure wouldn't tell them.

Sometimes Jennifer would not have even one bowel movement for three or four days. She'd sit on the toilet for an hour or more in the morning, even though it made her late for school. She could feel that the stool was there, but no matter how much she strained, it didn't come. Sometimes she couldn't even pass gas, which she also knew was there. She worried the gas would pass by itself, while she was in class or hanging around with her friends. The pressure that she always felt in her lower belly was made worse by the tight, low-slung jeans she liked to wear.

On other days Jennifer had diarrhea so badly that she had to run to the bathroom as many as ten times. By the end of the day only oily water came out. At school she had to use a stall in the girls' bathroom. The lack of privacy was horribly embarrassing. "I can't wait until there's no one in the bathroom," she said, blushing. "First because I can't wait, and second because there's always someone in there. And they can hear and smell everything." Jennifer often skipped school on the days she had diarrhea rather than face the girls' bathroom.

Jennifer should have been used to her digestive problems, because she'd had them for years. Her mother called Jennifer her "problem child" because she'd had a "nervous stomach" since she was a baby and had always been prone to diarrhea and constipation.

Jennifer had been to so many doctors that she knew beforehand what they are going to say. They couldn't find anything wrong. She just had a "sensitive stomach," and had to watch what she ate. But there wasn't a clear-cut relationship between what Jennifer ate and her symptoms. She didn't know what to watch *for*.

At 15, Jennifer went to see a specialist in intestinal conditions, a gastroenterologist. He didn't find anything wrong either, but he did have a name for her condition: irritable bowel syndrome, or IBS for short. He gave her a list of foods to avoid, including caffeine, sugar, chocolate, carbonated beverages, and red meat, among others. (There went burgers and sodas.) He told her to keep a diary to record what she ate, how much she ate, and when she ate, and what her bowel results were. "There's really not much else we can do," he told her. "You'll have to learn to live with it. And maybe it will get better in a few years."

A few years! To a teenager, a month is a long time, and a few years can seem like an eternity. Right now is what matters. The Junior Prom was coming up, and Tom, a boy Jennifer had had a crush on since eighth grade, had asked her to go with him. Jennifer was elated, but deep inside she was afraid. Worries chased around her head in an endless game of tag. What if she was bloated and fat and couldn't fit into her dress? What if she farted in the fancy restaurant he was sure to take her to? What if she had diarrhea and couldn't find the bathroom in time? Would he laugh at her? Would he be disgusted? She thought that maybe she should just cancel the date and forget about the Junior Prom altogether.

Carl

"Carl" had always been a healthy person, and at 32 he was at the peak of physical fitness. Not only was he in great shape, but all the areas of his life were going well. He was engaged to be married to a beautiful, intelligent woman he loved. He was already a middle manager in a Fortune 500 company, and all the signs pointed to a brilliant career as he moved further up the corporate ladder. He was the pride of his large, close-knit family, and he had plenty of good friends.

When Carl injured his knee playing touch football at the Fourth of July family picnic, he regarded it as "no big deal," even though the injury required surgery. Carl breezed through it with minimal pain and came home from the hospital the next day with prescriptions for antibiotics and pain meds, which he took even though he didn't really think he needed them. In just a few weeks he was walking without a limp and bragging that he was "as good as new."

Well, almost as good as new, except for the diarrhea that started right after he came home: explosive diarrhea, the kind that erupts — loudly — with very little warning. In the days right after his surgery, Carl couldn't get to the bathroom in time, and he soiled his pants more than once. Embarrassed, he scrubbed his pants out in the bathroom sink so his fiancée wouldn't see them.

The doctor didn't seem too worried. He gave Carl a prescription for Prilosec, a common acid blocker, but it didn't help. It wasn't unusual for Carl to visit the bathroom five or six times a day. When he returned to work, his frequent bathroom visits became a joke with his staff. Carl laughed with them, because he was a good sport, but inwardly he didn't find the situation amusing at all.

Carl's job required some travel, and business trips became a nightmare. He didn't always know where the bathrooms were in the places he visited. At conferences and meetings, he sat in the back so he could make a quick exit if he had to. When he and his boss made a road trip, driving over three hours to an outlying location, Carl had to ask his boss to stop at roadside gas stations three times. They were late to the meeting, and although his boss didn't say anything, Carl was sure he was irritated.

Carl's job also required him to give presentations, something he was good at and had loved to do — before the diarrhea. But now he worried he would have to rush from the room during a talk. He worried that his company would lose business if he embarrassed them. He stopped eating and drinking in the hours before a presentation — what didn't go in couldn't come out, he figured.

Months passed but Carl's diarrhea didn't. The doctor did some tests but couldn't find anything wrong with him. He said that stress was probably the culprit. After all, Carl had an executive job in a fast-paced industry, he was soon to be married, and he had recently had surgery — all big stress factors. The doctor recommended that Carl relax more. "Try to get out on the golf course more," he suggested.

Carl wondered if the doctor was really hearing him. He did enjoy golf, and would love to get out on the course more — but unless he installed a Port-o-Potty on his golf cart, Carl didn't see how golf could be an option.

Carl and his fiancée got married in a big church wedding, which went well despite Carl's fears that he would have to leave his bride at the altar while he rushed down the aisle looking for the church bathroom. They went to Hawaii on their honeymoon, but, although it was about the most relaxing place he had ever been, Carl's diarrhea did not abate. They had planned to go scuba diving, but Carl was afraid of having an attack out on the boat or in the water. So his new wife went scuba diving without him.

Carl had now had diarrhea for over a year. His family's traditional Fourth of July picnic was different this year, because Carl didn't come. In fact, he had skipped quite a few family functions over the past year. He missed them, but he worried that he wouldn't be able to control his bowels. "Why should I stink up their bathrooms, too?" is what he said to his wife the last time she suggested going to a family function.

Linda

"Linda" was 45 years old but said she felt more like 60. For much of her life she had suffered from constipation. She rarely had more than one bowel movement each week, and when she did her stool was tiny, round, and hard, like rabbit pellets. "It's been this way for so long I've forgotten that it isn't normal," she said. "When I found out some people pooped once a day, I thought *they* were sick."

In her thirties, Linda began suffering from intermittent severe abdominal pain. She would feel fine for a week or two, and then suddenly she would be stricken by cramps and stabbing pains in her lower abdomen for three to four days. She couldn't go to work or do anything else. The doctors could find no cause for the pain no matter how many tests they ran. All that they could suggest was that Linda watch her diet and limit her stress, and hopefully the pains would subside. In the meantime, they prescribed pain medications.

The medications gave Linda some relief, but the cramps and stabbing pains never left entirely. In fact, they grew more frequent. By the time she was in her forties, the pain had become Linda's constant companion. Now she was taking Vicodin (a powerful pain medication) every day, just to be able to function.

Linda was considering quitting her job as a fifth-grade teacher, even though she had always loved teaching, because she had less patience with the children than she used to. Although the Vicodin dulled her pain, she felt that the constant ache in her abdomen dragged her down. The noise and excitement generated by a room full of 10-year-olds seemed too much for her to take.

It was no better when she went home. Linda's teenage children complained that she was cranky all the time, and she knew they were right. Everything irritated her — their clothes, their music, their loud opinions. Sometimes she caught herself wishing they'd go away and leave her alone. Then guilt washed over her — how could she think that? She *loved* her children.

Linda's husband tried to be sympathetic, but Linda was sure that he too was tired of having a wife who was always fatigued, in pain, or fuzzy-minded from painkillers. She couldn't remember the last time they went out and had real fun together. They hadn't made love in months. Linda didn't blame her husband for his lack of interest. She didn't feel very sexy, and knew she didn't look sexy either. She felt old, and nothing seemed to give her joy anymore. Now menopausal symptoms had been added to her list of complaints. One of the last doctors Linda saw told her she had IBS and speculated that her symptoms might be due to menopause. If this is so, snorted Linda, it must be the longest menopause on record!

It's IBS

Even though their symptoms and circumstances differ, Jennifer, Carl, and Linda were all told they have the same condition: irritable bowel syndrome, or IBS.

Although the term *IBS* is fairly new, the condition has been around for a long time. It has also been called colitis or spastic colon, among other terms. In fact, poor digestion and the symptoms that make up IBS are more common than any other ailment known. Far too often these symptoms are accepted as normal. Or they are ignored because they are embarrassing to discuss. After all, your bowel movements are a private thing, not a subject for polite discussion.

IBS is not actually a disease, but a term used to describe the symptoms of poor digestive function. IBS can include abdominal pain, bloating, gas, heartburn, constipation, diarrhea, indigestion, or any combination of these. The symptoms may range from mild to severe and may be continuous or intermittent. As the stories of Jennifer, Carl, and Linda illustrate, IBS is not a trivial condition. It significantly affects everything you do, and can sometimes rule your life, robbing you of the enjoyment or contentment of your daily routine.

The diagnosis of IBS is usually one of exclusion. This means that the diagnosis is made after other serious conditions have been ruled out. In other words, if you don't have X, Y, or Z, you must have IBS!

If you have been given a diagnosis of IBS, you, like Jennifer, Carl, and Linda, were probably at first relieved to have a *name* for what was wrong with you. We like to have names for things. It makes us feel more in control. But wait a minute — IBS isn't really a *name*, it's just a description of symptoms. You already know your symptoms. So calling it IBS isn't really telling you anything new.

Jennifer, Carl, and Linda were each told there was no cure for their IBS. They were told to manage their condition, learn to cope with it, and accept it as part of their lives. Dietary changes, stress reduction, and medications were the tools recommended to help them manage, cope, and accept.

Remember, IBS is a description of symptoms. The tools used in IBS treatment can be effective only for relieving these symptoms. They cannot target the cause, because the cause has not yet been identified.

But what if there were a cause? What if the symptoms of IBS were due to physical abnormalities that could be treated *and cured?*

The stories of Jennifer, Carl, and Linda have happy endings. They are not still learning to manage, cope with, or accept their symptoms. They no longer live their lives in service to their intestines. Their bathrooms are no longer the most important rooms in their houses.

That's because they no longer have IBS. The causes of their symptoms were discovered and treated. They were cured. If you have been given a diagnosis of IBS, it is very likely that you can be cured too. This book explains how and why.

The fate of a nation has often depended upon the good or bad digestion of a prime minister.
— **Voltaire (Francois Marie Arouet),
French writer and philosopher (1694 – 1778)**

CHAPTER TWO

You Are Not Alone

IBS: More common than you'd think

You may be male or female; adult, adolescent, child, or infant; black, white, brown, or in between; from America, Europe, Africa, or Asia — and you may be diagnosed with IBS. If you have chronic symptoms of constipation, diarrhea, gas, bloating, or abdominal pain, you are not alone.

It is estimated that 20% of people worldwide suffer from IBS. While 25 million is a conservative estimate of the number of IBS sufferers in the US, most estimates are over 50 million. This means that nearly one in five people in America is suffering from diarrhea, constipation, bloating, or abdominal pain on a regular basis. You know how much you suffer when you have these symptoms. Now multiply your suffering by 50 million. That's how much intestinal distress is "out there" at any given moment.

Physicians see approximately 3.5 million patients a year with IBS, which accounts for 12% of all diagnoses in primary care medicine; nearly 30% of people who visit a gastroenterologist, a doctor who specializes in digestive diseases, are diagnosed with IBS. Despite this, studies show that 25% to 50% of Americans with IBS do not consult a physician. This isn't surprising, considering the lack of treatment options typically available for IBS.

IBS costs money

IBS is the second leading cause of worker absenteeism; only the common cold causes workers to use more sick days. The economic costs of IBS include hospitalizations, physician visits, missed work, and out-of-pocket expenses. Although these costs are somewhat difficult to quantify, the total cost of IBS in 1998 was reported to be $30 *billion* (not including medications). It has also been estimated that around $8 *billion* dollars a year is spent on medications, both prescription and over-the-counter, to combat the symptoms of IBS.

Who gets IBS?

Culture and gender

In the United States, women report symptoms of IBS approximately four times more often than men. Women also seem to have more frequent and severe symptoms, which interfere more with their daily activities. The American College of Gastroenterology reports that 80% of IBS sufferers in the US are women.

However, in other countries the opposite is true. In most parts of Asia, for example, the percentages are nearly reversed, with men being more likely to seek help for IBS symptoms. This may be because in other countries — unlike in America — men are more likely than women to go to the doctor.

Sociologists suggest that patterns learned in childhood may explain why women in Western cultures are more likely than men to report abdominal symptoms. Boys who are taught to "take it like a man" may grow up to be men who don't complain about something they see as trivial. Women are more likely to view IBS symptoms as a serious problem, whereas men often laugh off their symptoms. (They seem to find bathroom humor funnier too.)

Ultimately it seems that the apparent gender differences in IBS rates are due more to culture than to any real difference in the numbers of men and women who have the condition.

For both sexes, studies have shown that IBS appears to be more common in Western countries than in some developing countries, yet it is more common in rural Africa than in African cities. It is also more common among Asian Americans than among white or Hispanic Americans.

Native Americans and African Americans often suffer a genetic enzyme deficiency that causes lactose intolerance, the symptoms of which are similar to IBS. Often when an African American or Native American complains of diarrhea or abdominal pain, lactose intolerance is immediately thought to be the culprit. Many times nothing else is suspected, although it is now believed that many African Americans and Native Americans may actually be suffering from something else instead, something typically called IBS.

Age of onset

IBS can affect people at any age, although evidence suggests that it is more common in younger people than in older people, and there is a notable decline in IBS rates among people over 50. The average age of IBS onset is the late teens to early twenties, but it can start in childhood — even in infancy.

IBS in infants and children often isn't quite the same as in adults. This is particularly true with infants. Infants may express their IBS as colic, frequent crying, inability to sleep, or spitting up much more than usual. While children's IBS symptoms are similar to those of adults, healthcare practitioners are usually reluctant to put the IBS label on children until they are older. Children may also experience something called *encopresis*, another form of IBS. However, the potential causes of IBS, which are discussed later in this book, are the same for all ages. Whether an infant, child, adolescent, or adult, if you suffer from IBS or the symptoms of IBS and are known to not have a more serious condition, this book is for you.

Common, but not normal

IBS is so common that even animals have been diagnosed with it! Zookeepers have reported primates suffering from chronic diarrhea or constipation. Veterinarians treat many dogs with constipation, diarrhea, or excessive gas (anyone who owns a dog will recognize this one). Animals affected by these symptoms show the same kinds of reactions that humans do — they might become irritable, or tired and listless, or even depressed. These animals are suffering from IBS.

IBS is a syndrome, not a disease. Irritable bowel syndrome is the socially acceptable way to describe the collection of symptoms that irritate the bowel. Since these symptoms affect such an enormous number of people, from every race, culture, gender, age, and walk of life, one wonders what's really wrong. All of these people cannot be "abnormal," yet their digestive systems are functioning in an abnormal way.

What's going on down there in the digestive tract?

To eat is human, to digest divine.
Mark Twain, American author (1835 – 1910)

CHAPTER THREE

Your Miraculous Digestive Tube

What is normal, anyhow?

IBS is, by definition, a chronic condition. In other words, if you've been diagnosed with IBS, you've had these symptoms for a relatively long time. Although occasional bouts of indigestion are fairly normal, they should be very temporary. But if you have IBS, it may have been months or even years since your body has functioned the way it is supposed to.

Digestion should be the natural process of an exquisitely complex system that converts food into the materials needed for life: vitamins, minerals, fats, amino acids (proteins), and sugars (carbohydrates). From the average person's point of view, it is a relatively easy, even unremarkable process, something you take for granted. But from a medical viewpoint it is truly fascinating.

A lot happens between the time you eat a piece of food and the time the waste products leave your body. Most people are concerned only with the two parts of the digestive system that require some active participation on their part — the food going in and the waste coming out. The steps between these two poles are involuntary, and you probably don't pay a lot of attention to them. In fact, most people don't even know their own anatomy, and vaguely refer to the internal parts of the digestive system as the stomach, belly, gut, guts, or tummy.

If you've forgotten what it is to feel "normal" or if you're not sure how your digestive system works, the following is a brief refresher. Although it is simplified, it will lay the groundwork for understanding the causes and symptoms of IBS.

An overview of a healthy system

Think of your gastrointestinal tract as a long, muscular tube. This tube starts at your mouth and ends at your anus, and, if you were to stretch it out to its full length, would be about thirty feet long with a surface area approximately the size of a tennis court. It is a highly specialized organ that is designed to do three very important things: convert food into something your cells can use for nourishment and then absorb it; protect you from invading organisms and toxins; and dispose of a large variety of waste products. It is truly amazing that these three vital functions are performed by one structure.

This tube is so specialized that it actually has its own nervous system, often called a second brain. It also has a significant defense system to protect it from outside threats; in fact, the largest part of our immune system resides in the lining of the digestive tract. And to top it all off, this tube contains a highly evolved ecosystem of organisms which are not only critical to proper digestive function, but which are also a vital part of the defense system. You can start to see that a problem in the digestive tract has the potential to indeed be a very big problem.

Technically, anything inside this tube is not really inside your body. When you ingest something, it does not go directly into the cells of your body. It goes into the tube. Once it has been processed and broken down, it either passes through the tissue wall of the tube or is sent on its way out of the body.

This tissue wall is a permeable "skin," similar in many respects to the one that protects you on your other exterior surfaces — the skin of your arms and legs, torso and face. Like your outer skin, the tube's tissue wall is protective, but it is also highly specialized for digestion and absorption.

Food moves down the tube by an involuntary process called *peristalsis*, a wavelike muscular contraction that carries the nutrients from top to bottom. This movement is controlled by the digestive tract's private nervous system.

The food breaks down into a number of substances as it moves down the tube in stages. Muscular valves close off portions of the tube while chemical processes are carried out at each stage. Different areas absorb different vitamins, nutrients, minerals, and even water. Substances necessary for digestion and absorption, including acids and enzymes, are secreted into different sections of the tube. Waste is also created at each step and moves down the tube toward the exit. All of these functions are highly coordinated, working together to provide you with proper nutrition and to protect you from harm.

Digestion in more detail

The digestive tract is an amazingly complex system. The following simplified diagram allows you to see its basic layout.

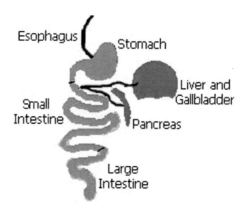

The process begins in the mouth, where your teeth break food down into more digestible bits. Step two is performed by the salivary glands, which produce digestive enzymes that also begin breaking down food. Swallowing is the next step and the last voluntary action before the food begins its journey through the tube.

After you swallow your food, it descends into the tube where involuntary processes take over. The food moves from the mouth to the pharynx, which pushes it downward into the esophagus. The food is then pushed into the stomach, which has a muscular valve at each end that keeps stomach acid inside the stomach where it belongs. (If acid escapes, you get heartburn.) The stomach churns the food and further breaks it down with acid, an enzyme, and other substances required for absorbing nutrients.

In two to six hours the food leaves the stomach in its new form and passes into the small intestine, where the cells lining the small intestine and secretions from the liver, gallbladder, and pancreas continue the digestive process. Most nutrients are absorbed in the small intestine. Whatever the small intestine doesn't break down or absorb passes into the large intestine, which contains the colon, rectum, and anal canal. Its major function is to absorb water and to pass undigested food and fecal matter out of the body.

The tube ends, of course, at the anus, where waste is eliminated by defecation. Here you again usually gain some measure of voluntary control, at least over the timing of elimination.

The ecosystem within us

Inside the digestive tube is a vast ecosystem where 100 *trillion* bacteria live. You should not be alarmed by this. We have been conditioned to think of bacteria as something bad, and the thought that we have 100 trillion "bugs" inhabiting our body can make us feel slightly queasy. However, although some bacteria are bad, others are very good. In fact, if you *don't* have them you feel very bad, because they are critical for proper digestion.

These bacteria have several important jobs: they help to break down food, they actually create some vitamins, they work directly with the immune system surrounding the digestive tract to protect us, and they independently protect us against invading organisms. Our relationship with the 100 trillion bacteria in our digestive tract has developed over hundreds of thousands of years. There should be no doubt about the importance of this ecosystem to good health.

The role of the immune system

The huge surface area of the tube must be protected against injury from bad bacteria, viruses, parasites, and other toxins that may get into the digestive system with food or by any number of other routes. The immune system is critically important in helping the intestines respond to these challenges. Possibly the greatest challenge to the digestive tract's immune system is to correctly tell the difference between what is bad (such as viruses and bad bacteria) and what is good (such as nutrients and good bacteria).

Your immune system must determine whether or not to develop a tolerance to everything you put into your mouth. Whenever you try a new food, it must decide, "Do I like this or do I attack and kill it?" You are always ingesting bacteria and other substances with your food, no matter how fresh and clean it is, so these must be screened out. While your immune system will "okay" most foods, genetic and other issues may affect its decision. Recent studies also suggest that your immune system's ability to develop correct tolerances depends a great deal on the balance of good bacteria inside your intestinal tract.

When you put something into your tube that the immune system doesn't like, it attacks by means of inflammation and excess mucus production. If your immune system is continually bombarded with messages to attack, its reactions can have major consequences. Inflammation of the digestive tube can in turn lead to damage of the lining of this tube, often resulting in something called "leaky gut" or "gut hyperpermeability." These two terms are simply descriptions of the damage to the digestive tract that is a result of something triggering an immune response. A severe example of this is a condition called celiac disease, which is caused by an intolerance to gluten. (Gluten intolerance is discussed in more detail in Chapter 6.)

Elimination

Elimination itself is fairly straightforward. Eating causes the colon to contract, beginning the process of peristalsis: contraction followed by relaxation, over and over again along the tube, moving things down to the exit. Between thirty to sixty minutes after eating (depending on various factors, such as how much was in the intestinal tract to begin with), a person will normally feel the urge to have a bowel movement.

About 60% of the fecal mass is made up of water, although this figure can vary widely. When you have diarrhea, for example, the percentage of water is much higher. About 30% of a normal stool consists of dead bacteria, which gives feces its characteristic odor. The rest is made up of indigestible fiber, fats (such as cholesterol), inorganic salts, live bacteria, dead cells and mucus from your intestinal lining, and protein.

Relaxation is a key to healthy bowel movements. In fact, the whole of digestive function is based on relaxation. This is why stress is often blamed for bad digestion. When you are relaxed, the parasympathetic part of your nervous system is dominant. This same part allows your digestive system to "do its thing."

Although the number of bowel movements a day that is considered "normal" varies, the average is one or two. Stools should be well formed; not watery; generally dark brown in color; and passed easily, without straining, cramping, or pain. Lighter brown stools, which usually float, generally mean you're not digesting fats very well. Ideally, at the end of the bowel movement you should feel like you are fully "through."

Evacuation is a fine balance and everyone is a little bit different, but the general rule is that if you experience discomfort, especially regularly, then things are not functioning normally. Pooping is a natural experience and should be comfortable and — dare we say it? — even bring an enjoyable feeling of release.

However, everyone, not just those diagnosed with a disease or IBS, will at times experience diarrhea, constipation, or excess gas. These symptoms, which vary in different people, can be caused by a variety of factors. What is happening in your body when these symptoms occur?

Diarrhea

The word *diarrhea* is derived from the Greek word *diarrhein*, meaning 'to flow through.' Basically, diarrhea is characterized by frequent, watery bowel movements. As you might suspect, diarrhea indicates that too much water is being retained (and therefore is not being absorbed) in the digestive tract.

There are several possible causes for this. For example, food may be moving through the tube too quickly for water to be absorbed, creating stools that are watery instead of formed. This can happen if your muscular tube starts contracting faster than normal as a defense against something bad that you've eaten. The immune system signals to the tube that it should get the bad stuff out quickly. It can go up or down, whichever is faster. If it goes up, you vomit. If it goes down, you have diarrhea.

Another cause is an immune response that leads to irritation or inflammation of the intestines. This can slow the absorption of water through the tissue walls, causing an imbalance in the tube's water level. Toxins in the tube can also cause water to flow into the tube rather than being absorbed. Any of these problems will result in diarrhea.

When you have diarrhea, you are losing water that would normally be absorbed. Therefore you are at risk for becoming dehydrated. Dehydration is a serious condition that affects every aspect of health and it is important to continue taking in fluids and seek medical help if you have chronic diarrhea.

Diarrhea also results in the poor absorption of nutrients including minerals, vitamins, proteins, fats, and carbohydrates. Each of these is essential to good health. Without them your body cannot function properly. Even if your weight is normal, if you have chronic diarrhea then you have a problem absorbing nutrients, and your health is being compromised. You should have not only the cause of your diarrhea, but also any potential nutrient deficiencies, evaluated.

Constipation

The two major factors for defining constipation are the frequency of bowel movements and their firmness. One sign that your digestive system is functioning optimally is that you have at least one bowel movement per day. However, bowel movements that are difficult to pass, very firm, or made up of small rabbit-like pellets qualify as constipation, even if they occur every day. Other symptoms related to constipation can include bloating, distension, abdominal pain, or a sense of incomplete emptying.

If you don't have these symptoms but you rely on extra fiber (such as Metamucil), a stool softener, a laxative, or some other method to prevent these symptoms, then you have constipation.

Constipation is a symptom of slow transit time, not unlike rush-hour traffic. When the colon is backed up, the small intestine is also backed up. And when the intestines are backed up, the stomach can be delayed in emptying itself of food matter. This is why some people with constipation also experience heartburn and reflux.

Constipation of course affects digestion and therefore can contribute to the malabsorption of nutrients, which can lead to a wide spectrum of health problems. It can also delay the removal of waste from the body, and not just from the colon. The liver is responsible for removing a majority of toxins (including pollutants, hormones, drugs, heavy metals, and even cholesterol) from the blood stream. Much of this waste is then dumped into the gastrointestinal tract for final disposal. If the tube is slowed in its transit time, then these toxins are not removed in a timely manner and may even be reabsorbed. This is akin to setting the garbage out at the curb but not having it picked up for several weeks. It's not good for the neighborhood, so to speak.

Constipation may also be painful. As fecal material passes through the intestine, water is absorbed out of it. The longer it remains inside the tube, the drier and harder to pass it will be, causing painful stretching of the colon as well as the anus.

There are essentially two different kinds of constipation. In the first type, the lower intestine cramps and spasms, like a charley-horse, and stops the fecal material dead in its tracks. If you could invite a masseuse into your lower intestine, that might help, and abdominal massage often does improve movement. But most people rely on other methods to relax the muscles, such as laxatives or stress reduction. Usually by the time it all gets moving again, the fecal material is hard and dry and painful to pass, causing a good deal of straining.

In the other kind of constipation, the lower intestine gets lazy and relaxes too much. This often happens when you rely on laxatives for too long. The digestive system comes to depend on the laxatives and your muscles lose their tone, becoming sluggish and unable to move fecal material along in the normal manner. This is typical of chronic constipation. Fortunately you can regain muscle tone over time, once the cause of the constipation has been found.

Gas and Bloating

One of the by-products of the breaking down of food is gas. Bacteria and digestion create some gas, which collects into bubbles and is expelled as flatulence. This is normal. However, if you are producing so much gas that it affects your social activity, or if the gas is especially odorous, then your body may not be breaking down food properly.

These symptoms of diarrhea, constipation, gas, bloating, and abdominal pain occur for an identifiable reason. They are caused by something that is not working the way it was designed to work. What could be causing this wonderfully efficient system to malfunction like this?

Digestion, of all the bodily functions, is the one which exercises the greatest influence on the mental state of an individual.
**Jean-Anthelme Brillat-Savarin,
French food author (1755 – 1826)**

CHAPTER FOUR

What's in a Name?

What does an IBS diagnosis mean?

IBS is called a diagnosis of exclusion, meaning that the diagnosis is made when other illnesses or conditions that may cause similar symptoms have been ruled out. These symptoms can occur for many other reasons, some relatively benign and trivial, some rare and serious. A physician needs to rule out the possibility that a serious health condition is behind the symptoms. But it is important to know that in the vast majority of cases, these symptoms, while they negatively affect your life, do not threaten it. In fact, being given a diagnosis of IBS implies that the physician has no idea what is causing your problem.

Feeling bad: The IBS experience

Most people will ignore a temporary or rare bout of diarrhea, constipation, or abdominal pain, expecting it to resolve itself within a short time — which it often does. But if you have had these uncomfortable or painful symptoms for a long while, or if they seem to come and go without warning, then you're probably pretty sick of feeling this way and would like to find out what's going on.

One thing that makes IBS so interesting is that its symptoms are highly individual. Some people suffer from diarrhea only, others have constipation, and in others diarrhea is followed by constipation or vice versa. Some have abdominal pain combined with diarrhea and/or constipation; others have only abdominal pain. The combinations of symptoms are as individual as the people affected.

One consistency among IBS sufferers is that the timing or quality of bowel movements is irregular. If you don't have at least one well-formed, easy-to-pass bowel movement per day, without doing anything special to your diet, then your digestive system is not normal. Irregularities you may experience if you have IBS symptoms include having fewer than one or more than three bowel movements a day. Your stool may vary in size or consistency; that is, it may be hard, pellet-like, pencil-thin, or loose and watery. You may have to strain to pass the stool, or you may experience a violent urge to have a bowel movement. In addition, even after a bowel movement you may feel that your bowels are not completely empty. You may feel bloated and your abdomen may be distended, or you may feel cramping or even sharp stabbing pains in the abdomen. Or you can feel any combination of the above.

Along with changes in bowel movements, you may also experience excessive flatulence, nausea and vomiting, loss of appetite, indigestion or heartburn, bad breath, prolific burping, mucus in the stools, or even symptoms not immediately related to the intestines, such as fatigue or headaches.

Whatever your list of symptoms, it is likely that they have persisted over a long time. You may experience symptoms off and on for many years, although they may be considered a chronic problem after as little as three weeks. The pattern of symptoms may change; you may go months without having any symptoms, your symptoms may recur many times a month, or they may be almost constant. Sometimes your symptoms may seem worse if you are under unusual stress. Sometimes your symptoms may seem worse after you eat. Or you may receive immediate, if temporary, relief from your symptoms after having a bowel movement.

By any definition, these symptoms are a pain. So you go to the doctor and ask, "What's going on?"

Plenty of unlikely causes

The doctor will first look for physical abnormalities. Modern medicine is very good at this. The doctor will ask for a complete medical history, perform a physical exam, and perhaps do laboratory tests or diagnostic tests such as x-rays, a colonoscopy, or an endoscopy. Because many serious conditions, including (but not limited to) colon cancer, endometriosis, ovarian cancer, and gallstones, can have the same symptoms as IBS, they must be conclusively eliminated as possible causes.

One condition often confused with IBS, because of their similar names, is inflammatory bowel disease (IBD), also known as Crohn's disease or ulcerative colitis. The symptoms for IBD include recurrent diarrhea (often bloody), cramping, abdominal pain, low-grade fever, and sometimes nausea and vomiting. IBD is far less common than IBS, but it is a serious medical condition. Interestingly, it can be caused by the same things that cause IBS.

There is a long list of other conditions that could be the cause of IBS-type symptoms. These include (in alphabetical order): AIDS; anal fissures; celiac disease; cirrhosis of the liver; congenital impediments; diabetes; diverticulitis; gallstones; gastroesophageal reflux disease (also known as GERD or acid reflux disease); hemorrhoids; hyperthyroidism; hypothyroidism; intestinal obstructions; lactose intolerance; lead poisoning (and poisoning by other toxins); multiple sclerosis; parasitical or bacterial infestation such as *Salmonella*; tuberculosis; ulcers; and on and on. It is fair to say that when you are sick, your intestines will probably let you know it.

Modern medicine is skilled in discovering these pathological conditions. Fortunately, most of these disorders are relatively uncommon, especially when compared with IBS, which affects 50 million Americans. And although some conditions are serious, the majority are treatable.

Lifestyles and life events may also lead to IBS-like symptoms. Lack of exercise or not drinking enough fluids can lead to constipation, for instance. Sudden changes in diet, such as a too-high intake of fiber or drinking excess coffee, may also cause a change in your bowel patterns, as will alcohol abuse.

Surgery or radiation treatments can give rise to constipation or diarrhea. Abdominal surgery, including hysterectomy, as well as other forms of abdominal trauma, can cause IBS-like symptoms due to the formation of scar tissue that adheres to the walls of the intestine.

Medications, both prescription and over-the-counter drugs, may be another source of IBS-type symptoms. Reactions to drugs are highly individual, as some people tolerate a given drug well, suffering no side effects, while others will suffer severe side effects. For this reason, it is especially important for your doctor to know your medical history. If you recently began taking beta-blockers for high blood pressure, for instance, and you have suddenly developed diarrhea, the medication may be the culprit. The following is a partial list of drugs that are known to cause IBS-type symptoms in some people: ACE inhibitors; beta-blockers such as atenolol; antibiotics like penicillins or ciprofloxacin; chemotherapy drugs; proton pump inhibitors such as Prevacid, Prilosec, AcipHex, and Nexium; nonsteroidal anti-inflammatory drugs such as Advil, Aleve, aspirin, Bayer, Excedrin, ibuprofen, Motrin, and naproxen; opiate analgesics; calcium channel blockers; antidepressants with anticholinergic effects; and even antacids and laxatives. You should not discontinue medications without talking with your doctor first.

Labs, scans, scopes, and other fun stuff

It should be clear that it is important to get yourself checked out for any of the conditions mentioned above. Simply put, a correct diagnosis can save your life. Depending on the severity of your symptoms, how long you've had them, your medical history, and observations from your physical exam, your doctor may order some tests to aid in your diagnosis.

Routine tests often include blood tests, stool analysis, and flexible sigmoidoscopy. Thyroid function tests are occasionally done. If the diagnosis is still unclear, further tests such as a colonoscopy, upper endoscopy, ultrasound, barium enema, or an upper gastrointestinal (UGI) series may be performed. If warranted, an abdominal computed tomography (CT) scan may also be ordered.

The vast majority of people with symptoms of consistent or recurring diarrhea, constipation, and abdominal pain pass these tests with flying colors. And even if something is found, it is often unrelated to their IBS. Most of them do not have colon cancer, gallstones, IBD, or any other condition from the long list above. And, although they are delighted when they're told they do not have a physical abnormality, they're also puzzled. Aren't diarrhea, constipation, and abdominal pain physical symptoms? Well, yes, but in their case there is no visible problem.

So these people are given a diagnosis that simply tells them something they already knew — their bowels are irritating them.

IBS: Doctors know what it isn't

According to the American College of Gastroenterology, IBS is defined not by what it is, but by what it is *not*:

- It is not an anatomical or a structural problem.
- It is not an identifiable physical or chemical disorder.
- It is not cancer and will not cause cancer.
- It is not a cause of other gastrointestinal diseases.

This is why IBS has sometimes been called the "garbage pail" disease. It is the diagnosis that remains when doctors feel that everything else has been eliminated. Most doctors have to define IBS this way because they do not know, or have not yet recognized, the cause of IBS. So what they are left with is a collection of symptoms.

When pressed to name a cause for IBS, most doctors have been trained to think of it as an illness that is more mental than physical, or an ailment that is primarily a gut reaction to life situations. They offer no cure for the condition. Treatment, if indeed any is offered, is at best palliative. That is, it aims to suppress or alleviate only the symptoms. Since IBS is viewed as having no identifiable cause, it is difficult for doctors to conceive of a cure. You may even be blamed for causing your IBS. Medications and lifestyle changes may be recommended, but you are offered no hope for a full recovery.

Unfortunately, just treating the symptoms, while sometimes helpful in the short term, is ineffective in the long term. It may even do more harm than good.

How's that working for you?

**Dr. Phil McGraw,
clinical psychologist (1950 –)**

*History teaches us that men and nations
behave wisely once they have exhausted all
other alternatives.*

**Abba Eban, Israeli foreign minister
(1915 – 2002)**

CHAPTER FIVE

Treating the Symptoms, Ignoring the Cause

Relieving symptoms

If you've been diagnosed with IBS, chances are you have been told that IBS cannot be cured. You've probably been told that you have to learn to live with the symptoms, try to control them, and manage your life around them. You may have been given various methods of managing your IBS. The three most popular are dietary changes, stress reduction, and medication. Probably you've been told to use a combination of all three.

When you are suffering from diarrhea, constipation, or abdominal pain, relieving these uncomfortable symptoms at the very earliest opportunity probably seems like a great idea. But while relieving your symptoms is of course important, these methods only work for the short term. They address and may alleviate your symptoms, but they do not cure IBS. And at their worst they may create more problems than they solve.

Before discussing the actual causes and cures of IBS in the next chapter, let's look at the benefits and challenges of using dietary changes, stress reduction, and medication to relieve symptoms.

Dietary changes and fiber

Although few physicians are trained to recognize food allergies or intolerances as a cause of IBS, they commonly agree that certain foods may trigger IBS symptoms. However, they do not necessarily agree upon which foods are wrong for which people, in what amounts sufferers should eat these foods, and when they should or should not eat them.

If you've done much reading about IBS diets, then you've seen advice urging you to decrease carbohydrates, decrease fats, increase fiber if you're constipated, increase fiber if you have diarrhea, cut back on sugar, drink more water, avoid lactose, avoid dairy, avoid bread, avoid red meat, cut back on yeast, reduce spicy foods, cut back on carbonated drinks and artificial sweeteners, eliminate chocolate, eliminate caffeine, eliminate alcohol, eat smaller meals, and so on and so on. You may be wondering if you can ever eat again without triggering your symptoms.

The problem with this approach is that different foods trigger IBS in different people, and many foods can potentially trigger IBS symptoms. The best diet for you may not be the best one for someone else. Certainly some people have been helped by one of the recommendations above. You may be one of those people, but then maybe you aren't.

Ideally, to create an optimal IBS diet, all you'd have to do is avoid a certain food or food group to discover whether it was triggering your IBS. Unfortunately this is easier said than done. It takes a great deal of time, persistence, and education to properly construct a diet that will adequately treat IBS.

Elimination diets

If you feel better after you've eliminated a food or stopped eating altogether, then you might strongly suspect that your diet is involved. You may have gone on a fast or a cleansing diet, or simply avoided food for a day or two and discovered that your IBS was much better. Of course, eventually you have to eat, and the trick is figuring out exactly what you *can* eat.

The purpose of an elimination diet is to identify whether or not specific food groups trigger your IBS symptoms. Essentially, during an elimination diet, you stop eating the foods you normally eat until your symptoms improve. You then slowly reintroduce your regular foods. If, when you reintroduce a food, your symptoms return, then it's likely that the food or one of its ingredients is an IBS trigger for you.

Before going on an elimination diet, you may be told to keep a food diary for a few weeks to log what you eat, when you eat it, and when you symptoms appear. However, the relationship between your symptoms, what you eat, and when you eat it is not always clear-cut.

For example, you may react to more than one food. In fact, most people with IBS are sensitive to more than one food or food group. You may suspect that your symptoms are caused by a certain food, but find that, even after you eliminate that food, your symptoms remain. This may lead you to mistakenly see the eliminated food as "safe."

Many IBS sufferers experience alternating constipation and diarrhea, which can be due to reactions to two different foods. One food reaction is causing constipation, while the other is causing diarrhea. These two foods are probably eaten fairly regularly and often simultaneously, making it very difficult to tie the symptoms to the food.

To find out if your diet is causing your symptoms, you may need to simultaneously eliminate virtually everything that you currently eat. This means that during the elimination diet you can eat only those foods that you do not currently eat. (Of course, it's also possible that you are intolerant to one of those foods as well.) If you avoid only one food group at a time, you may feel a little better but still not have the complete solution to your IBS diet problem.

Several factors make elimination diets difficult. For example, if you eliminate your regular foods during the diet, what *do* you eat? Some elimination diets are undertaken while eating foods that are supposedly hypoallergenic, such as lamb, pears, or rice. Unfortunately, selecting foods to eat during an elimination diet is complicated, since you can be intolerant to any food — including lamb, pears, or even rice.

During an elimination diet, you must stay away from entire food groups, not just one or two foods. Food groups are much more difficult to avoid than you might think. For instance, wheat, barley, and rye are related grains that all contain a protein called gluten, which is a major cause of IBS. Gluten is found in all foods made from one of these three grains, including most breakfast cereals; virtually all bread products including white bread; pasta; cookies; cakes; soy sauce; pancakes; waffles; some soups; and many other foods.

Another food group that commonly causes problems for IBS sufferers is dairy. Dairy is not just milk. Dairy includes cheese, butter, sour cream, cream cheese, ice cream, and yogurt. It's found in many baked goods such as muffins, breads, and cookies, as well as in many cream soups, some salad dressings, and milk chocolate. Even margarine contains dairy.

Two key components of dairy are whey and casein, which many people cannot tolerate. These are used as additives in a great variety of foods, even those you wouldn't consider to be dairy foods. Look at the labels on the packaged or processed foods you buy. Even non-dairy coffee creamer contains casein, for instance.

These examples show how complicated it can be to avoid entire food groups in order to assess the dietary trigger of your symptoms. If you remove only one part of a food group from your diet, you won't really know if that group actually causes your symptoms. You need a great deal of information about the foods you eat and what they contain in order to understand which foods trigger your symptoms.

Time is another factor that complicates an elimination diet. Usually, elimination diets must be followed for extended periods of time — several days or even weeks — before your symptoms improve. You must avoid all foods that are common to your normal diet for at least two weeks before reintroducing them. You should then reintroduce only one new food every three days, because food reactions may not show up for one to two days. If you add too many foods at once, you will not know which one triggered your symptoms.

The quantity of food you eat is yet another factor. If your body is intolerant to a particular food, a tiny speck of it may be enough to trigger symptoms. For example, cutting out your regular glass of milk is not enough to determine whether or not dairy is the cause of your problem. Unless you have eliminated every dairy product from your diet, as well as all supposedly non-dairy products that contain dairy components such as whey and casein, you may never really know.

A better and far easier way to determine how food is affecting you is discussed in Chapter 8: Stop Guessing!

Fiber

Increasing fiber intake seems to be the most popular treatment for IBS. Fiber can be soluble, meaning that it partially dissolves in water, or insoluble, meaning that it doesn't. Although neither type cures IBS, soluble fiber (which is also called viscous fiber, and is found in foods such as oatmeal, okra, or legumes, such as garbanzo beans) can be helpful in treating IBS symptoms, especially constipation and diarrhea. Insoluble fiber is more of a "scratchy" fiber; it adds bulk to the stool. A good example of insoluble fiber is celery.

Basically, fiber moves bulk through the intestines and helps to balance the pH (acidity) level in the intestines. It also helps to keep healthy the good bacteria that live in your digestive tract (see Chapter 7). In particular, one type of plant fiber, fructooligosaccharide (FOS), feeds these good bacteria. FOS is discussed in more detail in Chapter 7.

Soluble fiber forms a thick gel that helps to properly form the stool in the digestive tract and move it through the bowel; it also adds bulk to the stool. Because it slows the stool's transit time, it helps to prevent diarrhea. Soluble fiber also prevents constipation, because the colon becomes filled with gel, as opposed to being clenched tightly around dry, hard stools.

The USDA recommends that adults take in a minimum of 25 to 35 grams of fiber daily, and soluble fiber should account for one-third to one-half of the total. As many as 60 grams of fiber per day is required for optimal health. If you eat at least five servings of fruits and vegetables as well as at least five servings of grain products per day, you are very likely meeting your fiber requirements. Unfortunately, the typical American eats only 10 to 15 grams of fiber daily.

> **One serving of vegetable is 1/2 cup cooked vegetable or 1 cup of a raw leafy vegetable (like spinach).**
>
> **One serving of fruit is one medium-sized apple/ or pear, or 1/5 cup berries.**
>
> **One serving of grain is 1/2 cup cooked grain.**

Most foods that are high in fiber have a mix of both soluble and insoluble fiber. Because the average diet contains three times as much insoluble as soluble fiber, it is best to focus on foods that are higher in soluble fiber. These include grains such as pasta, oatmeal, rice, and soy; vegetables such as potatoes, carrots, and yams; and fruits such as bananas, papayas, and avocados.

The problem, however, with recommending a generic list of high-fiber foods is that individuals may have an intolerance to one or more of them. If you have a problem with soy, wheat, gluten, or the like, then increasing your consumption of these foods may actually make your symptoms worse.

Commercially available fiber products are simply concentrated forms of the fiber found in foods. They include Metamucil, Konsyl, Citrucel, Fiberall, FiberCon, Equalactin, and Benefiber. Metamucil, Konsyl, and Fiberall contain psyllium, which is often effective. However, some people find that it makes their symptoms worse.

Fiber is a good thing. Taking extra fiber, either through food or products such as Metamucil, can help to alleviate your symptoms. However, it is very unlikely that your diet is so low in fiber that a deficiency is actually the cause of your symptoms.

Therefore, fiber is not the ultimate solution to IBS.

Supplements and digestive aids

Supplements are often marketed to those with IBS. They include vitamins, minerals, digestive enzymes, aloe, betaine HCL, butyrate, fennel, and glutamine, among others. People with IBS are searching for answers, and many of them are willing to try almost anything in that search for help. But the fact is that all of the supplements and digestive aids in the world are unlikely to cure your IBS. This is because, except in special cases, the cause of your IBS is not likely to be a supplement deficiency.

However, many supplements do have beneficial properties that can help heal the digestive tract and optimize digestion, especially once the true cause of the problem is addressed. A range of very high-quality digestive supplements is available at **www.ibstreatmentcenter.com**.

The bottom line about diet

The biggest problem with the traditional dietary change approach to IBS is that it is too generic. Not all IBS sufferers have problems with dairy, for instance. Not all IBS sufferers get sick when they have a glass of wine. Not all IBS sufferers are helped by adding extra fiber to their diet. This approach is not targeted toward individuals. It views food as the problem, instead of recognizing that the problem lies within each person's response to food. And each person is unique.

Stress reduction

Most physicians are trained to think of IBS as stress induced or as a type of psychosomatic disorder. Because physicians have not been able to diagnose the causes of IBS or cure it, IBS has been framed in a way that suggests that it is more your problem than the physician's.

It has been stated that people with IBS tend to have more anxiety about their health and to seek medical attention more often than others. It has also been suggested that these people have been programmed to behave as if they are ill. Early studies showed that psychiatric disorders and psychiatric symptoms occurred three times more frequently among patients with IBS than among patients with gastrointestinal conditions of a "known organic cause." Anxiety and depression were the most common psychiatric symptoms, but other conditions such as phobias, obsessive behavior, sleep disturbance, panic attacks, and hostile feeling were also more common in IBS patients.

Although some cases of IBS are no doubt related to mental or emotional issues, and stress and anxiety can aggravate IBS (as it can most other medical conditions), these are not the predominant causes of IBS. Although several causes, discussed in more detail later in this book, have been discovered, medicine has focused primarily on emotional issues as the cause of IBS. Unfortunately, the fact that treatments based on other causes have been successful continues to be viewed by many health care practitioners as merely due to the fact that the patients believe they will work, and therefore irrelevant to medical treatment.

Medicine has a long history of blaming medical conditions with no known organic cause on some form of psychological disturbance, such as stress — only to discover later the organic cause of the problem. One excellent recent example of this is stomach ulcers. While stomach ulcers were once thought to be a stress-induced disorder, it is now well accepted that they are caused by the bacteria *Helicobacter pylori*. In many cases the discovery of the organic source of a problem is made long before this knowledge is commonly used in the standard of medical practice. Sometimes this delay is even decades long.

It is true that stress can make the symptoms of IBS worse, and that your digestive system depends on relaxation to function properly. Occasionally stress *is* the sole cause of IBS. But your chronic diarrhea or constipation will itself cause you stress! And, believe it or not, the problem that is causing your IBS may also cause anxiety or even depression.

If you have been diagnosed with IBS, it is likely that you have been advised to reduce your stress level. You may have been told to get regular exercise and adequate sleep, and to practice stress reduction techniques such as yoga, meditation, tai chi, deep breathing, journal writing, relaxation therapy, biofeedback, hypnotherapy, or psychotherapy.

All of these practices can indeed improve physical, mental, and emotional health. They provide a host of benefits, from improved personal relationships to enhanced productivity to increased energy and mental clarity, and they just might help with your IBS symptoms.

But chances are they won't cure your IBS.

Medication

At least 20 million Americans have been diagnosed with IBS. The drug companies are beginning to tap into this hefty target market by offering medicines aimed at relieving the symptoms of IBS. These drugs alter the physiology and ultimately the action of the digestive tract, but they do not address the underlying causes of IBS, or even claim to cure IBS. These drugs also come with an alarming variety of warnings and side effects.

Six types of drugs are used to treat the different symptoms of IBS. They include the following:

- IBS-specific drugs to control the speed with which the bowels move (Zelnorm, Lotronex, and Calmactin),

- laxatives to treat constipation (such as Milk of Magnesia, Ex-Lax, Perdiem, and MiraLax),

- antidiarrheal agents to treat diarrhea (such as Imodium and Lomotil),

- antispasmodics to relive the pain from abdominal cramps (such as Donnatal, Levsin, Levbid, NuLev, Bentyl, and Pro-Banthine),

- antidepressants to relieve pain (such as Prozac, Celexa, Zoloft, Paxil, and Elavil), and

- narcotic analgesics to relieve pain (such as Vicodin, Demerol, and Xanax).

Note that these drugs are categorized by the type of symptom that they treat. However, what may be useful for one symptom may make another worse. For example, antidiarrheal agents may relieve diarrhea at the cost of worsening abdominal pain and bloating. Constipation may be relieved by dietary fiber or bulk laxatives, but patients frequently experience an increase in bloating and abdominal pain that makes the treatment unacceptable. Abdominal pain may be dulled temporarily by antispasmodics, but these drugs can cause constipation, and the pain may return with increased intensity. Antidepressants and narcotic analgesics may dull the pain of IBS, but they certainly don't address the cause. In addition, many IBS patients are intolerant to drugs of any sort because they make their symptoms worse.

These drugs change how you experience IBS by forcing changes in the biochemistry of your body. None is capable of curing IBS, because IBS is not caused by a drug deficiency. Treatment with these drugs does not address the cause of your IBS, and once you stop using the drugs the symptoms will return. As discussed below, the use of these drugs often results in serious side effects and/or negative long-term consequences.

IBS-specific drugs (Zelnorm, Lotronex, and Calmactin)

IBS-specific drugs, such as Zelnorm, Lotronex, and Calmactin, are relatively new. They change your symptoms by changing the motility (muscular action) of your digestive tract and by altering your sensation of pain. Some of them inhibit motility and slow transit time, and are therefore used for treating diarrhea. Others stimulate motility and decrease transit time and are therefore used for treating constipation. They do not cure IBS.

Zelnorm is used to treat constipation. It changes the normal biochemistry of the digestive tract and stimulates it to increase motility and thus increases the movement of stool through the bowel.

Lotronex was removed from the market in November 2000, due to potential side effects. In June 2002, Lotronex was again approved by the US Food and Drug Administration (FDA) to treat IBS-related constipation in women. It is approved only for short-term use.

In April 2004, the FDA issued a warning that Zelnorm has been associated with serious cases of diarrhea, as well as with instances of ischemic colitis, a potentially deadly medical condition in which blood flow to the intestines is reduced. In the new warning, the FDA stated that serious complications from diarrhea had been reported both during clinical trials and after Zelnorm was put on the market. These included significant loss of fluid, low blood pressure, and episodes of passing out. In some cases, patients had to be hospitalized for rehydration.

The FDA thus recommended that Zelnorm not be used in patients who have diarrhea or are prone to it. If you are taking Zelnorm and you develop low blood pressure, lightheadedness, dizziness, or fainting spells, you should stop taking the drug and contact your doctor immediately.

The agency also said that patients who develop symptoms of ischemic colitis, such as rectal bleeding, bloody diarrhea, or new or worsening abdominal pain, should stop using the Zelnorm immediately. You should be tested for ischemic colitis and should not take Zelnorm again if there is an indication that you might have this condition.

Zelnorm was designed only for short-term use in women. It is not known whether it is safe and effective for men. Potential additional side effects from taking Zelnorm include headache, leg or back pain, and joint pain.

Lotronex, which is used to treat diarrhea, also changes the normal biochemistry of the digestive tract, but in exactly the opposite manner to Zelnorm. Lotronex inhibits motility and slows the movement of stool through the bowel.

Lotronex was approved by the FDA in February 2000 for use in women with IBS-related diarrhea. However, it was withdrawn from the market in November 2000, when life-threatening side effects, including ischemic colitis, were associated with its use. In June 2002, the FDA again approved the drug, and it became available in November 2002.

This time, however, the FDA imposed restrictions on its marketing. Lotronex can be prescribed only by doctors who are considered qualified to recognize and manage IBS; these doctors must enroll in a special prescribing program. It can be used only by women who have severe diarrhea associated with IBS. In addition, patients must be educated about the risks associated with the drug.

Calmactin is a drug for diarrhea-predominant IBS that is currently undergoing clinical trials and may be out by the publication date of this book. Similar to Lotronex, Calmactin inhibits intestinal motility and slows transit time.

Again, these drugs do not cure IBS.

Laxatives for constipation (includes Milk of Magnesia, Ex-Lax, Perdiem, and MiraLax)

Different laxatives work in different ways, but all essentially increase the amount of water in the bowel and thus lead to a softer stool. Many people use laxatives every day, and become dependent on them to move their bowels. Laxatives do not cure IBS, and should be used only temporarily while finding the cause of the problem. Before starting the use of laxatives, you should determine whether you can improve your constipation by taking a non-prescription soluble fiber supplement, drinking lots of fresh water, and increasing exercise.

There are three main classes of laxatives: osmotic laxatives, stimulant laxatives, and emollients.

Osmotic laxatives are intentionally designed to be poorly absorbed. By changing the digestive tract's normal biochemistry, they cause water to enter the small intestine and colon, thus softening the stool. The most common compounds used in laxatives are magnesium and phosphate. One well-known brand is Milk of Magnesia. Others include Uro-Mag, Citroma, Fleet Phospho-soda, and K-Phos Neutral tablets.

Osmotic laxatives can be made from other compounds. For example, MiraLax is a nonabsorbable laxative made from polyethylene glycol. It does not contain magnesium or phosphate. Laxatives made from polyethylene glycol typically cause less gas, bloating, and flatulence than those made from other compounds.

Sorbitol and lactulose are also used to make nonabsorbable laxatives. Intestinal bacteria partially breaks them down into compounds that cause water to collect in the colon. This results in softer stools. Sorbitol and lactulose can, however, still cause flatulence, bloating, and cramping. Sorbitol products include Mirilax, Cystosol, Resulax, and Sorbilax. Lactulose products include Enulose, Cephulac, Kristalose, and Duphalac.

Osmotic laxatives, especially when they are used too much, can have serious complications, including severe diarrhea and dehydration. Because they can also cause electrolyte disorders, people with kidney or heart disease should be closely monitored when using them.

Stimulant laxatives irritate the bowel wall, increasing muscle contractions and motility. There are two main classes of stimulant laxatives: diphenylmethane derivatives such as Dulcolax and Correctol, and conjugated anthraquinone derivatives such as senna (Ex-Lax, Perdiem and Senokot are senna-based laxatives), cascara sagrada, alder buckthorn, rhubarb root, yellow dock, and aloe vera. Castor oil is a third type of stimulant laxative; it acts in the small intestine rather than in the bowel.

Complications associated with stimulant laxatives include dehydration and electrolyte disturbances. Castor oil can cause cramps and diarrhea. As with all laxatives, you may over time become more and more dependent on them for moving your bowels.

Emollients soften the stool in one of two ways. Docusates allow it to absorb more water and oil, while mineral oil simply adds oil to it. Emollients do not cause as many side effects as other types of laxatives, but they are also generally less effective.

A docusate is basically a detergent that is not absorbed by the body. It lowers the surface tension of the stool, which lets water and fat pass into the stool. It does not hold water like some bulking agents, nor does it stimulate the bowel like many laxatives. Two brands of docusates are Colace and Peri-Colace.

Mineral oil (one brand is Fleet Mineral Oil) coats the bowel and stool, trapping moisture within the stool, which softens it and makes it easier to pass. When taken orally, mineral oil can be dangerous to patients who have difficulty swallowing, because if it is inhaled into the lungs it can cause pneumonia.

Laxatives do not cure IBS.

Drugs for diarrhea (includes Imodium and Lomotil)

There are essentially three types of drugs used for treating diarrhea in IBS, those that coat the digestive tract, those that bind to receptors in the intestine and those that bind bile acids. You do not need to understand either of these mechanisms, but they help us to categorize these antidiarrheal medications.

The first type and the most common over-the-counter medications for diarrhea are Pepto-Bismol and Kaopectate. The drugs sooth the digestive tract by coating it with bismuth, and they also have slight analgesic properties somewhat similar to aspirin. Since 2004, the FDA has recommended that antidiarrheals containing bismuth subsalicylate, including Pepto-Bismol and Kaopectate, not be given to children under 12 without a doctor's instructions. In fact, the FDA required that dosing information for children under 12 be removed from the labels of these products.

The second type of antidiarrheal includes brands such as Pepto Diarrhea, Imodium, Lomotil and Lomocot. These are the drugs the interact with receptors in the intestine. They improve the absorption of water in the intestine, strengthen the tone of the anal sphincter, and decrease bowel transit time, therefore reducing the frequency of bowel movements. These drugs are designed to be taken before meals or events that normally trigger a patient's IBS symptoms.

These drugs are chemically related to narcotics and can be habit forming. Because Imodium and Pepto Diarrhea (not to be confused with Pepto-Bismol) do not cross the blood-brain barrier, they are not as likely to become as addictive as Lomotil and Lomocot, which do cross the blood-brain barrier. Since an overdose could be fatal, you should take only the recommended dose, and you should be especially careful in giving these drugs to children. These drugs also can cause constipation. You should discontinue using them if the constipation becomes severe.

Antidiarrheals containing cholestyramine, such as Questran and Cholybar, attempt to stop diarrhea by binding bile acids. When the transit time through the small intestine is rapid, bile acids are poorly absorbed; this can lead to diarrhea. Some people have found that these types of antidiarrheals are helpful after gallbladder surgery, although clinical studies have not yet confirmed this.

These drugs do not cure diarrhea or IBS.

Antispasmodics for pain (includes Donnatal, Levsin, Levbid, NuLev, Bentyl, and Pro-Banthine)

Antispasmodics are possibly the most frequently prescribed drugs for IBS pain. They discourage muscle contractions (and thus spasms) in the digestive tract by blocking normal nerve activity and inhibiting certain nerve impulses. The two forms of antispasmodics available in the US are anticholinergics and peppermint oil.

Anticholinergics come in several different forms and under a number of brand names. Some examples are Levsin, Levbid, NuLev; Bentyl, Bemote; Pro-Banthine; Librax, Clindex; and Donnatal.

These drugs have a range of side effects. The most common are dizziness, blurred vision, headaches, difficulty urinating, a decrease in sweating, rashes, itching, and dry mouth, nose, throat, or skin. Other potential side effects include constipation; bloating; nausea; vomiting; fever; clumsiness; unsteadiness; fainting; fatigue; drowsiness; trouble sleeping; memory loss; confusion; a false sense of well-being; hallucinations; unusual excitement, nervousness, restlessness, or irritability; increased sensitivity to light; eye pain; decreased flow of breast milk; irritation at place of injection; warmth and flushing of skin; muscle weakness; slurred speech; difficulty in swallowing; difficulty in breathing; fast heartbeat; and convulsions

Peppermint oil prevents calcium from entering into the cells of intestinal muscles. This inhibits muscle contraction and relaxes the intestinal muscles. Although side effect from peppermint oil are rare, they can include slow heartbeat, heart-burn, nausea, headaches, rashes, muscle tremors, and loss of muscle coordination. Nausea and heartburn can be decreased or prevented by taking peppermint oil tablets that are enteric coated, such as Elanco. The coating slows the rate at which the tablets dissolve.

Antispasmodics, including peppermint oil, do not cure IBS.

Antidepressants for pain (includes Prozac, Celexa, Zoloft, Paxil, and Elavil)

Antidepressants are often used in the treatment of chronic pain associated with IBS. They can raise the patient's pain threshold for abdominal cramps by changing the normal biochemistry of the nervous system in the digestive tract. Two classes of antidepressants used by IBS sufferers are tricyclic antidepressants (TCAs) and selective serotonin reuptake inhibitors (SSRIs). In addition, because they affect the rate of muscle contraction in the digestive tract, they can be helpful in the treatment of diarrhea or constipation.

However, antidepressants can potentially worsen IBS symptoms such as diarrhea, constipation, and pain, depending on the patient and on the class of the drug. SSRIs (such as Prozac, Celexa, Zoloft, and Paxil) can increase the rate of muscle contraction in the digestive tract and can trigger severe IBS attacks in patients who suffer from diarrhea. TCAs (such as Elavil and Norpramin) decrease muscle contraction and may make constipation worse.

Antidepressants come with a variety of potential side effects. The most common side effects associated with SSRI-type antidepressants are nausea, headaches, insomnia, and sexual dysfunction. TCAs can cause sedation, increased appetite, urinary retention, blurred vision, and constipation. TCAs are especially dangerous for the elderly, who may experience confusion, delirium, or loss of balance.

Antidepressants do not cure IBS.

Narcotic analgesics for pain (includes Vicodin, Demerol, and Xanax)

Narcotic analgesics are either opiate drugs (made from opium or one of its derivatives) or opioid drugs (having an effect similar to opiates, although not containing opium). The most effective painkillers available, they work by depressing selective parts of the central nervous system. They also cause drowsiness and a feeling of tranquility. Narcotic analgesics are addictive; therefore they should be used only when needed and not on a regular basis.

Common narcotic analgesics include Vicodin, Demerol, morphine, Darvocet-N, Xanax, Valium, and Ambien. The most common side effects of these medications are sedation, dizziness, light-headedness, nausea, and vomiting. In addition, these drugs may cause drowsiness, anxiety, fear, restlessness, mood changes, confusion, decreased mental capabilities, blood disorders, constipation, difficulty urinating, decreased physical capabilities, hearing loss, rashes, itching, slowed breathing, and sluggishness.

Narcotic analgesics do not cure IBS.

More trouble than help

A study published in the *Journal of Clinical Gastroenterology* in October 2004 reported that side effects from taking IBS drugs are extremely common. Nearly 75% of the IBS patients surveyed reported that they had to discontinue drug-based treatments due to side effects. Many of them also sought medical help or missed work, school, or social activities because of the side effects. This once again leads us to the obvious – these drugs don't cure IBS.

Ignoring the causes

Dietary changes, stress reduction, and IBS medications all focus on alleviating IBS symptoms, period. They cannot cure IBS, because in order to cure, you first must know the cause. And this search for the cause is exactly what is missing in the current evaluation and treatment of IBS.

Yet there is a cause. Current research and clinical evidence indicate that there are three main causes of IBS symptoms: food allergies, bacterial imbalances, and parasites.

There are many reasons that most doctors don't recognize food allergies or a bacterial imbalance as a cause of IBS. Doctors are a product of their education, and their education does not focus on or often even address diet, nutrition, good bacteria, or the complex ecosystem in your digestive tract. Most doctors assume that, unless you have a serious allergic reaction to a given food, food is generally good for you. They believe that most dietary issues are related to either calories or exercise.

There is a significant amount of research to counter this attitude, but it has yet to be taken seriously, and it gets lost in the vastness of medical research. A large university medical library will have several thousand different scientific journal titles, which contain hundreds of thousands of articles. You might assume that all scientific information gets put to good use, but the fact is there is way too much of it for that to be the case, and as of yet there is no way to properly assimilate all of it so that one person, or even one organization, can understand and use it. Medical students, doctors, and institutions must decide to focus their efforts only on what they feel is most important for learning or teaching.

Also, physicians are rewarded for doing things the way they've always been done. This is what being a good physician is all about: memorize everything to perfection and then apply it. In medical practice this is called the "standard of practice." There are few incentives to go beyond the standard of practice, and in fact, going outside of the standard of practice is likely to draw the wrath of peers, professional associations, and certainly insurance companies.

Most importantly, medicine is a business, a fact that many people easily forget. The pharmaceutical industry spends a tremendous amount of money to influence the field of medicine, in obvious ways such as advertising in medical journals, and in not so obvious ways such as giving physicians financial incentives to prescribe their medications. Even health insurance companies are given incentives by pharmaceutical companies to promote certain drugs over others. As well, physicians make more money by doing complex procedures than by talking with and educating patients. The result is that the assessment and treatment methods chosen are often those that provide the greatest profit margin, not necessarily the greatest benefit to the patient.

Physicians are generally good people and go into medicine for all of the right reasons. But they sometimes get lost in the complex world of the business of health care, where it can be extremely difficult to keep one's distance from or even recognize these issues.

Ultimately, we are a free market society, and there really is no financial incentive to cure problems. Once a problem is cured, it is gone. It is much more profitable to create a long-term situation that requires long-term care. This may sound cynical, but it's just common business sense.

So most medical practitioners continue to treat the symptoms and remain ignorant of the true causes of IBS. They are victims of their own system, which does not let them see that there may be a cure.

This is unfortunate, because the majority of IBS sufferers can be cured of IBS, completely. There is no need to be the victim of an incurable diagnosis.

PART TWO

The IBS Solution

What is food to one may be fierce poison to others.

**Lucretius, Roman Epicurean poet,
philosopher, and scientist
(c. 99 B.C–c. 55 B.C.).**

CHAPTER SIX

Is It Food or Is It Toxic?

Food allergies: A true cause of IBS

Food isn't supposed to be toxic, right? But if you're allergic to a particular food, that's exactly what it is. Food allergies may be one of the most prevalent health problems in America. Some studies indicate that over two-thirds of those diagnosed with IBS suffer from negative reactions to the food they eat. Recent and ongoing studies suggest this figure may be considerably higher.

There is increasing evidence that food allergies and intolerances are more common and have a greater impact on our health than previously realized. Some experts estimate that future research will show nearly 50% of the population has some sort of food allergy or intolerance. This is not as unlikely as it seems.

To illustrate, one area that has been intensely researched is celiac disease, which is caused by an intolerance to one specific protein, gluten. (Gluten is a component of many grains, including wheat.) Nearly 1% of the population (3 million Americans) suffers from an intolerance to gluten.

That's just one protein, not even an entire food! With that in mind, it doesn't seem so unreasonable that half of the US is suffering from a food allergy or intolerance. It would certainly explain a lot of health problems. (See Appendix A.)

Who, me?

If you're like most people, you're probably thinking, "Not me, I don't have an allergy." Most people think they have a pretty good understanding of food allergies. They may know someone who has one and think, "My problem isn't like theirs." Or they may think that food allergies normally result in hives, a rash, or some kind of medical emergency.

However, food allergies can cause many other health problems, such as IBS. Inflammation is a consequence of an allergy, and inflammation is responsible for many conditions, from sinusitis to joint pain. Also, studies have clearly shown that food allergies interfere with the absorption of nutrients. This can also result in significant health problems, the most obvious being osteoporosis due to decreased calcium absorption, and iron deficiency anemia due to poor iron absorption. In some cases food allergies do not cause major symptoms until one of these chronic diseases shows up later in life.

You might have a tough time believing that you may have a food allergy, because you've eaten the "offending" foods before, some every day, and have not suffered from severe symptoms. Maybe you've had just a little diarrhea or constipation once in a while, until suddenly it gets worse or new symptoms develop. Symptoms of food allergies, including IBS symptoms, can show up at any age, from birth to old age. Why they show up when they do is still unknown, but, if you have an intolerance or allergy, you've probably had it all your life.

Even if you've never suffered from it before, over time it will catch up with you. The body is amazing in its ability to adapt to a variety of conditions and stresses. However, eventually your body will be dealing with so many issues that negatively affect your health that it can no longer hold out and symptoms will start to appear. It's like filling a bucket with water. You can keep pouring more water in until it reaches the top, but eventually it's going to spill over and cause a problem. Each person has a unique threshold at which he or she experiences symptoms, depending on genetic inheritance, environmental issues, and all of the other factors that affect his or her health.

Holly

At 33, Holly had her first child. Deciding to stay home with the baby for a year or two, she quit her job to become a full-time mother. Although she loved being home with her daughter every day, she had one problem.

A year after the baby's birth, Holly still had not lost the twenty pounds she had gained during pregnancy. She knew why, too. Dealing with the demands of an active toddler, Holly found it just too difficult to fix herself a regular breakfast and lunch. Making the family dinner was as much as she could manage. Instead she relied on snacks — usually cookies, potato chips, and other high-calorie goodies.

Holly finally joined a weight-loss program that helped her get back onto a better eating program. Although she didn't give up snacking, she replaced the cookies and dough-nuts with celery sticks, apple slices, and a few handfuls of almonds for protein.

The weight loss program worked. In six months, Holly had lost her excess weight and looked great.

But she didn't feel great. For months she had suffered from nausea, bloating, and gas attacks that embarrassed her even when the only one witnessing them was her baby daughter. She also complained of fatigue, backache, and insomnia.

Holly's doctor could find nothing wrong, even after a full GI investigation. All he could suggest was that her problems were caused by the stresses of being a mother, and he advised her to find a babysitter so she could get some time for herself.

When Holly's symptoms persisted, she came to the IBS Treatment Center, where she was tested for food allergies. The tests were negative for all foods except one — almonds! Her favorite high-protein snack was having more of an effect on her than she realized.

Holly began snacking on cashews instead of almonds and in two weeks all her IBS symptoms had disappeared.

Allergy versus intolerance

You may have heard the word *intolerance* used in addition to or instead of *allergy*. The words *food allergy* and *food intolerance* are often misunderstood and misused. They can even cause confusion among doctors and other members of the medical community. Although they are sometimes used interchangeably, they really refer to two different things. Therefore it is important that we define these two types of reactions to food.

Allergies and intolerances are two distinct types of physiological events. With an *allergy*, the body's immune system attacks something that it shouldn't. However, an *intolerance* doesn't arise from the immune system at all. This is the key difference between the two, so let's explore it in greater detail.

Allergy

Allergies are reactions that involve the immune system. Food should not normally trigger an immune response. Unfortunately all too often it does, and the immune system produces antibodies that target the food. Antibodies in turn trigger inflammation, which can result in pain and tissue damage, leading to further symptoms. Excess mucous production can be another product of an immune response.

When a food triggers an immune response, the antibodies circulate throughout the body. This is why an allergic reaction can be exhibited in such a variety of symptoms just about anywhere in the body. (See Appendix A for a list of these symptoms.)

However, it is not really understood why an allergy is expressed so differently in different people. Each individual seems to have a unique weak point where symptoms show up first. In many people that point is somewhere in their intestinal system and therefore they wind up with IBS.

Intolerance

A food intolerance is any type of non-immune reaction to or problem with a food. The most common example is a digestive enzyme deficiency, such as with lactose intolerance, in which a person cannot properly digest milk products. Lactose intolerance is the most common food intolerance in America, affecting as many as 30% of adults. It is an intolerance, not an allergy, because the person is either deficient in or lacks the enzyme lactase, which is needed to break down lactose in the small intestine. If lactose is not broken down, it will pass into the large intestine, where it may cause flatulence, diarrhea, or other symptoms.

Many people believe they have lactose intolerance when actually they have a dairy allergy, or both lactose intolerance and a dairy allergy. They cannot drink milk or ingest any milk products without "paying for it" later, just like someone who does have lactose intolerance. But what is happening inside them is very different.

Many people suffer from stomach pain or heartburn after eating spicy food. Although this can be caused by an allergy, in most cases it is simply a negative reaction to hot, spicy foods, another type of intolerance. This reaction does not appear to be an enzyme deficiency. Other intolerances include reactions to preservatives (such as sulfites and nitrites), colorants (FD&C colors), and flavorants (such as monosodium glutamate/MSG and aspartame). Medically speaking, we classify these poorly understood reactions to foods or food additives as intolerances.

IgE and IgG: Two important allergic reactions

IgE and IgG are acronyms for two different kinds of antibodies produced by the immune system in allergic reactions to food. You might be asking why you need to know this. The reason is that conventional allergy testing at best only tests for one of these antibodies and not the other, which means that you do not get the whole picture from traditional allergy tests. As a result, many people who do have food allergies don't know that they do.

The immune system is very complex, and is still not totally understood. But basically, it functions like a sentinel standing guard against foreign invaders. One weapon it uses against invaders (in the case of an allergy, the invaders are called *allergens*) is the production of antibodies. The antibodies cause reactions that result in the offending allergens being removed from the body.

The immune system produces numerous kinds of antibodies, called immunoglobulins, which is what the *Ig* stands for. (The *E* or *G* designator signifies particular kinds of antibodies.) Conventional allergy testing looks for IgE reactions only. These types of reactions typically occur immediately after contact with or ingestion of the allergen, and in some cases can cause serious, even fatal, health problems. Potential IgE reactions include swelling of the lips and tongue, hives, bloating, abdominal pain, or sudden diarrhea. These are the reactions that people usually think of when they hear the word *allergy*. However, IgE reactions can also lead to many other symptoms not traditionally recognized as being caused by food allergies.

The problem is that most food allergies are not IgE, but are rather IgG reactions, which usually show up hours or even days after ingestion of the allergen. They are generally not nearly as dramatic as the more severe IgE reactions, and usually result in "mere" constipation, diarrhea, bloating, water retention, fatigue, eczema, and so on. However, as we have seen, IBS and other symptoms, when left unrecognized and untreated, not only destroy quality of life, they can lead to chronic and debilitating "dis-ease."

Skin testing versus blood testing

For several decades skin testing has been the standard way to test for allergies. The potential allergen is injected under or scratched into the skin, and any resulting inflammation (also known as *wheal*) is measured. The size of the wheal determines whether or not an allergy is diagnosed. This technique leaves a lot to be desired because we don't inject food into our skin when we eat, nor do we necessarily get a red bump when we have a food allergy. Equally important, this test can measure only an IgE antibody reaction. And even then, you may have high levels of the IgE antibody in your blood, indicating the cause of your IBS, and still not get a positive skin reaction. The IgG antibody is not tested for at all.

Many people are incorrectly told after skin testing that they do not have a particular food allergy. Others seem to react to everything that is tested. Skin testing is probably relevant only for life threatening (anaphylactic) types of food allergies, but in these cases the patient often already knows that he or she has the food allergy.

A more accurate way to detect most food allergies is through ELISA (ee-LIE-za) testing of the blood. This test measures the actual amount of both IgE and IgG in the blood. ELISA stands for Enzyme Linked Immunosorbent Assay, a big, fancy phrase for a laboratory procedure in which antibodies are detected and measured. This very specialized procedure is performed only by doctors trained in recognizing and treating food allergies. It is run only by specialized labs equipped to handle such sophisticated testing, and *accurately* run only by those labs that have strict quality control standards.

For the patient, testing involves a simple blood draw. The blood is then sent to the lab and any antibodies against food that are present in the blood are detected and measured. A typical food allergy panel measures reactions to approximately 100 of the most common foods found in the American diet (listed in Appendix B). The test is a direct measurement of the immune system's response to food. It is not affected by what the patient ate on the day of the test. In someone with no food allergies, no antibodies will be detected. However, in a very high percentage of people with IBS symptoms, this test uncovers elevated antibodies to a specific food or foods.

Invariably, these people feel better after removing the offending food or foods from their diet.

The testing procedure will be discussed in more detail in Chapter 8.

Why do people have food allergies?

There are many theories about why people develop food allergies, and there are probably several causes. One theory is that an allergic person's immune system did not develop properly, for reasons not totally understood. A baby's immune system develops as the baby is exposed to different foods. The immune system learns what is good for the health of the body, and what is not. If a food is not good for the body, the attack system goes on alert to wipe out the offender. An allergy results when the immune system makes a mistake, identifying a food as bad and reacting accordingly.

Most food allergies are probably due, at least in part, to genetic inheritance. People in the same family often suffer from the same health problems. Because allergies often run in families, it is common to find that parents, grandparents, and children produce antibodies to the same foods. Although people may be aware that their symptoms are similar to those of their relatives, they don't always realize there is a food allergy triggering those symptoms, and that if they avoid the food then they can avoid the symptoms. You don't always have to suffer just because Mom, Dad, Grandma, or Grandpa does.

Allergies may also occur due to the fact that throughout most of human history, many present-day foods were not part of our natural diet. Therefore we did not necessarily evolve to accept them all as nutrition. This may be why so many people have problems with the same types of food. For example, an allergy to dairy, or products made with cow's milk, is the most common allergy of all. Dairy was not a staple of the "cave man" diet, as animal husbandry is a recent innovation. We haven't all been fortunate enough to get a body that recognizes dairy (or many other foods) as nutrition. It's sad, but true.

Immune responses may also be learned in infancy, if the mother is allergic and breastfeeding, since she will pass on her antibodies to her baby in the breast milk. The baby will then react to the antibodies and may exhibit symptoms, whether or not the mother does. The baby may also react to the foods the mother is eating, and even if she is not allergic to that food, the baby might be.

Regardless of the cause of food allergies, when it comes to food we are not created equal. Many of us just simply cannot eat certain foods without a negative consequence.

Those sneaky foods

Why is it so difficult to detect your own food allergy? The difficulty is in connecting the symptoms with your eating habits. You eat every day, yet your symptoms seem to vary in intensity, or they come and go altogether. Often you don't associate the problem with the food because the feedback isn't immediate, or because you are eating the food too often. Perhaps you don't make the connection between the symptoms and the food because you don't eat much of that food. Even if you eat something only once or twice a week, it may be causing significant symptoms throughout the week.

The timing of an allergic reaction can vary widely. It can take place immediately or up to three days after eating an offending food, and it can last anywhere from thirty minutes to several days. By that time you have eaten a variety of other foods, so without a blood test it is nearly impossible to tell which foods are causing your reactions.

Further complicating the matter is that a given food does not necessarily cause the same symptoms in different people. For example, cheese may cause some people to become constipated, but other people may react with diarrhea or abdominal pain. The amount of food eaten may also affect the intensity of the symptoms in some people but not in others. For some people, a tiny hidden amount of a food may fully trigger their symptoms. Others seem able to tolerate small amounts, but experience symptoms with larger amounts.

Any given symptom can be caused by a number of different foods. For example, one person may have constipation due to dairy products, another due to eggs, and another due to wheat. It is also true that many people have multiple food allergies with multiple, overlapping symptoms. Any food at all has the potential to be an allergen. This is why the elimination diets discussed in the previous chapter are often difficult to undertake accurately and are frequently unsuccessful.

Finally, the foods we eat are not always straightforward. Foods may include additives, preservatives, or ingredients that you may not recognize as your particular allergen. If you are allergic to eggs, for example, it doesn't mean you'll react just to scrambled eggs at breakfast and egg-salad sandwiches at lunch. It means your immune system will recognize the egg in that egg pasta at dinner, too. And as for dessert — well, many baked goods also contain eggs. No wonder you don't feel better when you avoid only the obvious sources of eggs.

Similarly, the labels of packaged foods may list ingredients that are actually components of other foods, using words you may not recognize. A good example of this is casein, which is often used as an additive or filler. Casein is a protein found in cow's milk, but you may not recognize it as a potential trigger for a dairy allergy, even if you do read labels.

Stan

Stan had been suffering from alternating constipation and diarrhea for nearly all of his 30 years when he was finally diagnosed with celiac disease, a gluten intolerance. He was advised to remove all sources of wheat, barley, and rye from his diet. This wasn't easy for Stan, since he was particularly fond of bread and especially of pasta dishes.

However, he complied with his doctor's advice, and soon Stan's diarrhea was completely gone. That would have been worth giving up pasta for, if only his constipation had gone too. But it hadn't. It had become worse.

His doctor was puzzled when Stan reported that his constipation was an even bigger problem than before. As far as the doctor was concerned, they had found Stan's disease. He told Stan that the constipation would resolve itself in time.

When his constipation did not get better with time, Stan decided to try food allergy testing. Because the testing had a much broader focus, it was discovered that he was allergic to dairy as well as gluten.

Stan again revamped his diet, this time removing all forms of dairy. Within three days his bowel movements had become regular. Even though he no longer eats the pasta he used to love, his life is much happier and healthier.

The top ten

Dairy and eggs are by far the two most common food allergies across the US. However, one may be allergic or intolerant to any food, or to none at all. Some people even react to such supposedly innocuous foods as broccoli, spinach, or rice, although allergies to these foods are fairly rare.

Here is a list of the ten (actually eleven) most common food allergies:

1. dairy (including butter, cheese, and yogurt)
2. eggs
3. beef
4. lamb (yes, lamb!)
5. goat's milk
6. peanuts
7. almonds
8. gluten (wheat, barley, and rye)
9. garlic
10. bananas
11. soy

To illustrate the complexities of dealing with a food allergy, we will discuss two of the better researched food allergies in more detail: dairy and gluten.

Dairy

Dairy may be the most misunderstood food in our culture. It is often assumed to be high in nutritional value and even mandatory for good health. "Drink your milk!" we expect American mothers to tell their children. But the truth is that dairy, or cow's milk and products made from it, creates significant health problems for many people. In the big historical picture, humans have only recently introduced cow's milk into their diet, so it is not surprising that the immune system does not always recognize it as a friendly substance.

Like any food allergy, a dairy allergy is capable of triggering a wide array of symptoms. Some of the most common complaints in addition to IBS include ear infections in children, sinusitis, heartburn/reflux, acne, headaches, anxiety, fatigue, irritability, joint pain, poor growth, and frequent illness. (See Appendix A for a more complete list.)

Lactose intolerance is often confused with dairy allergy. As stated previously, lactose intolerance is not an allergy, but a deficiency in the enzyme lactase, which is the enzyme that digests the milk sugar lactose. However, lactose intolerance can be the result of a dairy allergy and the two can share the same symptoms — upset stomach, bloating, gas, and loose stools.

Many people say that taking Lactaid or a similar digestive product designed for lactose intolerance helps their problems. However, the fact that Lactaid is effective for them is not necessarily because they are inherently lactose intolerant. Rather, a food allergy may have damaged the digestive tract to the extent that it has caused a deficiency in lactase, which is produced by the cells lining the digestive tract. And Lactaid doesn't resolve other problems that can be caused by their food allergy.

Ear infections, especially in young children, are often a result of a dairy allergy. At first glance, the connection between ear infections and a dairy allergy is not clear. But the process is actually very simple. If a child has a dairy allergy, the allergy is likely to cause inflammation and blockage of the eustachian tube in the ear, which in young children is not fully developed. Children generally consume a lot of dairy, and it is commonly one of the first foods introduced into their diet. Removing dairy from the diet will usually result in ear infections becoming a thing of the past.

Dealing with a dairy allergy is a lot more complicated than most people think. If you have a dairy allergy, it may not be just milk that you are allergic to. You may be allergic to all dairy, including cheese, butter, sour cream, cream cheese, ice cream, and yogurt. But given the simple definition of *dairy* as anything made from cow's milk, it would seem fairly easy to identify foods that are made from it. However, in today's marketplace it just isn't that easy.

Dealing with processed and packaged foods, which form a significant part of the American diet, is complicated. Lactose, which is a primary sugar in cow's milk; casein, a primary protein in cow's milk; and whey, the watery part of cow's milk that separates from the curds, are all added to a wide variety of foods, including baked goods such as muffins, breads, and cookies, as well as cream soups, salad dressings, margarine, cereals, high-protein beverage powders, infant formulas, nutrition bars, whipped toppings, and milk chocolate. Even bakery glazes, breath mints, and non-dairy (!) creamers may contain either lactose or casein. You may not get better until you avoid everything made with dairy products.

Gluten

Gluten is a protein found in wheat, barley, and rye, and is responsible for the springiness and stretchiness of bread. Allergies and intolerances to gluten have been the subject of intensive research over the past decade. Much of this research has focused on celiac disease, which is a special form of gluten intolerance. It is a hereditary response to gluten that results in a very specific type of damage to the small intestine. Common symptoms, which can mirror those of IBS, include loose stools, constipation, or both; fatigue; weight fluctuation; dermatitis; and more.

The rate of celiac disease is much higher than previously thought. According to a recent study, 1 in every 133 people suffers from the disease, making it one of the most common genetic disorders known. Relatives of those with celiac disease are even more likely to have the disease themselves — 1 in 22 first-degree relatives (parents, children, or siblings), and 1 in 39 second-degree relatives (aunts, uncles, first cousins, or grandparents) will also test positive for the disease.

Celiac disease is commonly referred to as a gluten *intolerance* rather than an *allergy*, even though it is an immune reaction. It is diagnosed by measuring damage to the small intestine, either by blood testing or, traditionally, with a biopsy of the small intestine. A positive biopsy means that the villi, or small finger-like extensions of the intestinal lining, have been damaged; this is known as villous atrophy.

People with celiac disease will show a marked reduction in their villi, almost as if the villi have been worn off. Damage to the villi causes a dramatic reduction in the surface area of the small intestine, resulting in both poor digestion and the poor absorption of many nutrients.

Biopsies are done in a hospital on an outpatient basis, but require strong medication due to the invasiveness of the procedure. An endoscopy is performed, which involves a tube being placed into the mouth, down the esophagus, and past the stomach. A tissue sample can then be taken from the small intestine.

Celiac disease is not the only form of gluten intolerance or allergy. Although no studies have been done on the prevalence of other types of gluten allergy, it is certainly much higher than that of celiac disease alone. Many people react to gluten by producing elevated IgG antibodies, but they do not have damage to the small intestine. Their test results for celiac disease are negative. They become quite frustrated with traditional medicine, with its narrow definition of celiac disease, because they are told that their negative test results meant that they are not allergic to wheat, barley, or rye. Yet when they eat a piece of bread they become sick.

The treatment for celiac disease and for a gluten intolerance or allergy is identical. It means removing all sources of gluten from the diet. This is not an easy task, because so many of our foods contain gluten. Dietary counseling can make the job easier.

Gluten is found in nearly all bread products and all pastas, as well as in most breakfast cereals, cookies, muffins, cakes, soy sauce, pancakes, waffles, soups, sauces, and gravies. Beer, ale, lager, and stout contain gluten. Malt, malt extract, and caramel flavorings, which are used to add flavor to a wide variety of foods, contain gluten. Even some medications contain gluten!

Grains with no gluten, such as oats, have sometimes caused confusion because they have been known to cause the same symptoms. This is because oats are often handled by the same mills, processing plants, and grain elevators that handle wheat, barley, and rye. The resulting contamination of the oats is enough to readily trigger a gluten allergy.

The good news

A beneficial result of the research into celiac disease is that now many gluten-free breads, pastas, and other foods are on the market. Similarly, dairy-free foods are also available for those who suffer from dairy allergies. These foods can often be found in local health-food stories or online at one of the many gluten-free and dairy-free food retailers. The same is true for most other major food allergens, including egg, soy, corn, and nuts.

The question of whether you have a food allergy can be answered through proper testing, as discussed in Chapter 8. In many cases IBS is purely the result of a food allergy. Although you can't cure a food allergy, the good news is that you may be able to cure your IBS. Knowing what foods to avoid will put you in control of your symptoms and will allow you to live your life on your terms.

*Support bacteria — they're the only
culture some people have.*

Steven Wright, comedian (1955 –)

CHAPTER SEVEN

Bugs: The Good, the Bad, and the Ugly

Whose body is it?

Your body is not yours alone. You are sharing it with over 100 trillion bacteria. This fact makes many people uncomfortable. "I have *bugs* living inside me?" you may ask, aghast.

Yes, inside the orifices of your body, and primarily in your digestive tract, live an enormous number of bacteria — single-celled organisms that have colonized areas of your body and exist happily there, eating, growing, and multiplying. The average adult carries about three to four pounds of bacteria in his or her digestive tract. There are several hundred different species of bacteria inside you at any given moment, including many different strains of the same species.

This may alarm you, because we have been trained to view bacteria as the enemy. Over the last century, medicine has been driven by an antibacterial movement, which holds that one of the most important keys to health is the maintenance of a clean, even sterile, environment. This movement has been responsible for the eradication of many diseases that used to decimate populations on a regular basis, and we owe a huge debt of gratitude to these medical pioneers.

However, we are not sterile beings. Life just isn't like that. Bacteria are everywhere — in the air you breathe, the water you drink and bathe in, and on all the surfaces you touch. There is no escaping them. Bacteria were here on earth before humans were, and it's probable they will be here when we are not. Bacteria and human beings belong together because we evolved together. Our internal bacteria are actually critical to our health — so critical, in fact, that we cannot survive without them. They are fundamental to the development of our immune system, they help break down our food, and they even create nutrients that we need for good health.

The bacteria inside us form a teeming, busy ecosystem. Just like in any other ecosystem, its organisms must have food and they need space in which to live and grow. Every organism is interconnected with every other and with its host — you. Changing or harming one species will have repercussions on the other species and on the host itself. While we are used to thinking of the earth's ecosystems in this way, it may seem strange that these same principles govern our internal environments.

The bacteria inside your intestines form a diverse population. The numbers of each kind of bacteria change over time, depending on your age, your diet, your health, and your use of supplements or drugs. The bacteria that thrive adhere to the intestinal wall and use the semidigested food that is passing through your intestines.

Bacteria begin to colonize inside you from the time of your birth. Before birth, you have a sterile digestive tract, but during the birthing process infants pick up the bacteria living in the mother's vagina. Infants require bacteria to start their immune systems off correctly. Hopefully the mother has good bacteria in a healthy balance, because increasing evidence shows that the presence of certain good bacteria helps develop immune tolerance to food and decreases the incidence of food allergies and other health problems.

The good guys

Healthy people live in harmony with their "good" bacteria, or normal intestinal flora. This is called symbiosis. We provide the bacteria with a home and food, and in return they do some great things for us.

Although there are thousands of different bacteria, the best-known friendly bacteria are *Lactobacillus acidophilus* and *Bifidobacterium*. *Lactobacilli* are also the bacteria that change milk into yogurt, and they are present in acidophilus milk. *Bifidobacteria*, which have been shown to provide many health benefits, are particularly high in the intestines of breast-fed newborns. A healthy intestinal system has more of both these friendly bacteria than other, unfriendly bacteria.

Because they are among the first colonizers of the sterile digestive tracts of newborns, these beneficial bacteria prime the immune system of the digestive tract. A recent study found that formula-fed infants have a different balance of bacteria than breast-fed newborns. For this reason, formula-fed infants may be at higher risk for diarrhea and allergies than breast-fed babies. The study also showed that adding *Bifidobacteria* back into the diets of formula-fed newborns diminished the incidence of both diarrhea and constipation. The study concluded that the beneficial bacteria were important for the immune system's development of tolerance. As was discussed in the previous chapter, lack of tolerance often leads to food allergies and chronic inflammation.

Good bacteria have also been associated with lower rates of asthma, eczema, and hay fever. Infants and children with strong populations of good bacteria are far less likely to develop these conditions than those who lack adequate populations of good bacteria.

Beneficial bacteria also help to produce Vitamin K and many B vitamins during the digestive process. They enhance motility and the proper functioning of the intestinal tract by helping to break down food so our bodies can absorb the nutrients. They also help to break down other compounds like some drugs and plant materials.

One of the most important services good bacteria provide is preserving the correct balance of bacterial populations within the body. By their very presence they prevent the establishment and spread of "bad" bacteria and yeast, because harmful bacteria and yeast generally have no place to grow if friendly bacteria are thriving. You can never have too many of these great bacteria. They never do any harm; they do only good. It's impossible to "overdose" on them.

There are always some unfriendly bacteria present in your digestive tract, too. Many of these are considered normal flora, as long as their populations are smaller than those of the good bacteria. They become a problem only when this balance is upset.

An imbalance between good bacteria and bad bacteria, yeast, or parasites is called dysbiosis. Dysbiosis is a major cause of IBS.

The bad and the ugly

What makes bad bacteria bad? The worst bacteria (the ugly) either directly destroy tissue by feeding upon it or produce a toxin that destroys tissue. Other bacteria (the bad) react negatively to food, or are poor fermenters of food, creating IBS symptoms like gas and diarrhea. And some species of yeast and bacteria are bad simply because they take up space, thereby crowding out the good bacteria and depriving your body of all the health-giving benefits that friendly bacteria provide, resulting in the poor digestion of food and the poor absorption of nutrients.

The ugly bacteria are never regarded as normal flora within the body. They are not usually considered to be causes of IBS, but they do cause severe, often life-threatening, conditions. Ugly bacteria include *Salmonella*, *Shigella*, *Yersinia*, *Vibrio cholerae*, *Campylobacter*, and certain strains of *E. coli*. Just a tiny amount of the most virulent strains of bacteria in a person's body is enough to begin the process of infestation. The symptoms of these bacterial infections usually include severe watery diarrhea, which is often bloody. Some cause vomiting, muscular cramps, dehydration, and permanent intestinal damage. If untreated, they may even cause death. In short, they are nothing to fool around with. Luckily, the medical community is generally good at identifying and treating these kinds of bacterial infestations.

Less dangerous, but still unwelcome, are the bad bacteria, which include the Enterobacteriaceae family of *Citrobacter*, *Enterobacter*, *Klebsiella*, *Proteus*, and *Serratia*, as well as *Clostridium difficile* and *Pseudomonas*. At very low populations, these bacteria may be considered normal flora in the intestinal tract. However, being normal doesn't make them good. Each has been documented as causing IBS-type symptoms, and they often need to be eliminated. Unfortunately most doctors rarely test for them, since the symptoms they cause are usually not immediately dangerous. But, if a bad bacteria has managed to increase its population and gain territory in your intestinal tract, you may experience gas, bloating, abdominal pain, or loose stools. You're probably not dying, but you are very uncomfortable.

You may be surprised to learn that another bacteria considered normal flora is one strain of *E. coli*. Due to some recent well-publicized cases of *E. coli* infestation, the name itself now seems scary. Some types of E. coli are scary, but the strain of *E. coli* normally found in the intestines is not the toxic strain that causes bloody diarrhea and other symptoms. In fact, we all have *E. coli* living in our intestines.

The key is to keep it there in our intestines; you don't want it in your eyes or throat, or on your skin. *E. coli* is a normal component of feces, so when sewage overflows into rivers or lakes, it can contaminate them. Therefore water sources are tested for the presence of *E. coli.* in order to determine whether or not they have been contaminated.

The best protection from the bad and the ugly bacteria is having plenty of the good guys around. That, and washing your hands. Remember, bacteria — both bad and good — are everywhere around us. Nothing on earth is sterile. On almost everything you touch, bacterial life is going about its daily business. When you breathe, sit in a chair, touch a door handle, brush by a tree branch, step on the grass — anytime you come in contact with anything, with any portion of your body — you are probably collecting bacteria.

This is normal. It's supposed to be this way. The good bacteria keep up their end of our symbiotic relationship by protecting us from the bad ones.

IBS problems can occur if you don't have enough good bacteria, or if they are overcome by a particularly virulent bad bacteria. Then, when you pick up some bad bacteria, they are free to colonize. If there are not enough good bacteria to challenge them for territory, they can establish themselves firmly within your intestines. Colonies can survive for decades if not properly treated.

It is one of life's ironies that the treatment that gets rid of bad and ugly bacteria — antibiotics — is also the primary cause of the bacterial imbalance that leads to IBS. Antibiotics kill bacteria, both the bad ones that you want them to kill and the friendly ones. If you don't replenish your digestive tract with good bacteria, your system is wide open to be colonized by more bad bacteria and yeast. Think of it like an intestinal Wild West — without good bacteria, there's no law and there's land for the taking. The bad guys can run rampant. This creates an unsafe and unpleasant environment.

Antibiotics are not the only threat to good bacteria. Friendly bacteria may also be killed or their populations reduced by alcohol, cortisone, and chemotherapy, as well as by stress, and even by a poor diet. Whatever the reason, when your friendly bacteria are gone, the result is often IBS.

Angela

Angela, who is 21 years old, took antibiotics to clear up a painful bladder infection. A few days after she began taking them, she began suffering from constipation, something which had never troubled her before. After a week of straining and hard, painful bowel movements, Angela started to experiment with the off-the-shelf remedies available at the local drugstore. Over the next few weeks she took stool softeners, various fiber concoctions, and a variety of laxatives, but nothing worked. The long straining sessions in the bathroom and the hard stools continued, and in addition, Angela began to feel tired and irritable all the time. She shared an apartment with her older sister, and Angela's general grouchiness caused several serious arguments to flare up between them.

Angela's sister, who was studying to be a nutritionist, suggested that Angela be tested for bacterial imbalances. Angela took her advice, and the tests showed that although she had no bad bacteria present, she was deficient in friendly bacteria, and she had a flourishing crop of Candida albicans, *commonly called a yeast infection.*

"I thought yeast infections were only vaginal," said Angela. "I didn't know yeast could get into your intestines too."

Antifungal medication was prescribed for Angela, along with a course of probiotics to build up colonies of good bacteria to keep any future yeast at bay. Although Angela began to feel better right away, the doctor warned her that Candida *was a strong opponent and it might take a while to be rid of it.*

"Candida is a real pain," said Angela. "I wish I had been told about this possibility when I took the antibiotics in the first place, so I could have prevented this from happening at all."

Yeast, a.k.a. *Candida*

Yeast infections, or yeast overgrowth, are a common result of antibiotic use. Yeast is also considered normal flora at low populations, since it is often found in the digestive tract. However, remember that normal does not necessarily mean good. Yeast, especially the most common type called *Candida*, invades tissue and is a general irritant. Its growth inhibits the growth of good bacteria, and its life cycle produces the toxic effects of IBS symptoms in its host — you. *Candida* will take advantage of every opportunity it has to flourish. If your system has been wiped clean of friendly bacteria due to antibiotics (which do not kill yeast), *Candida* will likely pounce, either in your digestive tract or elsewhere in your body. Once it gets hold, it can be difficult to get rid of.

Candida can cause a huge variety of symptoms, including but not limited to all the symptoms of IBS, making it one of the most frustrating and confusing conditions to describe, not to mention endure. The average *Candida* sufferer reports about twenty different symptoms. Many sufferers give up trying to find out what is wrong with them because their symptoms seem unrelated. Diet can affect *Candida* symptoms too. Since yeast feeds upon sugars, a diet high in sweets, alcohol, starches, and refined carbohydrates may increase its growth. As a result, some health practitioners recommend special *Candida* diets that are low in sugar and refined carbohydrates.

If you think you may be suffering from a *Candida* infestation, it is very important that you undergo proper testing as soon as possible, as it can become a chronic condition if the fungus is allowed to take hold. If your tests are positive, you will be treated with the correct antifungal agents. The next chapter will explain the testing in more detail.

The best way to treat a yeast overgrowth is, of course, by preventing it in the first place. Make sure your friendly bacteria are well established, so that *Candida* has no chance to grow and spread. After using antibiotics, you should always replenish the intestines with good bacteria. How to do this is discussed at the end of this chapter.

Parasites

Parasites, another cause of IBS symptoms, can cause diarrhea, constipation, gas, bloating, cramps, nausea, poor digestion, fatigue, muscle aches, bleeding, rectal itching, and abdominal pain. Parasites cannot live without you. You provide them living space and food, but unlike friendly bacteria, parasites do nothing for you in return. They only act against you.

Parasites vary in size from the very tiny, which can be seen only under a microscope, to inches long. Some can find their way into just about any area of the body, but most are found only in the digestive tract. The severity of your symptoms and the amount of damage they cause varies depending on the parasite involved, the number of parasites, and the level of resistance your body has.

Parasites damage the body in a number of ways, by absorbing nutrients that you need and by directly damaging your digestive tract, and, if they are capable of migrating, possibly damaging other areas of your body as well. They often reproduce rapidly and by the thousands, and are easily spread to other people. Unfortunately, a strong population of good bacteria does little to protect you from parasites.

Parasites are more common than generally believed. Although most Americans consider them to be a Third-World problem, they infect millions of Americans — even those who never leave the country or drink from mountain streams (a common source of the parasite *Giardia*). We live in a global community. Parasites enter this country every day through the importation of contaminated foods and seemingly innocent products such as clay pottery. It is true that many common parasites are native to the tropics, where it is warm and humid. But the fruits and vegetables we import from these warm countries can be a source of parasitic contamination, affecting every area of the United States. However, because of the misperception that parasites are not an American problem, they have often been overlooked as a possible cause of digestive illnesses.

Entamoeba hystolytica, a relatively common parasite, infects up to 50 million people worldwide each year, and results in up to 100,000 deaths. In Dhaka, Bangladesh, approximately 50% of children have signs of exposure to this parasite by age five.

Closer to home, one of the largest recorded outbreaks of a waterborne parasitic infestation occurred in Milwaukee, Wisconsin, in 1993. The city's water supply became contaminated with the parasite *Cryptosporidium*, which causes diarrhea, abdominal cramps, and nausea. Over 400,000 people became ill; 4,000 were hospitalized and over 100 died. Although Milwaukee's water was treated with chlorine, chlorine doesn't kill *Cryptosporidium*.

There are two major categories of parasites: protozoa and worms. Protozoa include the one-celled microorganisms *Giardia*, *Entamoeba*, *Cryptosporidium*, and *Blastocystis*, which all live in the digestive tracts of their hosts, including humans. These four common parasites cause similar symptoms — most often diarrhea, but also fatigue, abdominal cramps, nausea, and other digestive ills. They are found worldwide and in every region of the United States. They are spread when the feces of infected individuals finds its way into food and water sources. Because these parasites are often spread as cysts, protected by an outer shell, they can survive outside the body for a long time, which makes them resistant to chlorination and some other water treatments.

Worms include roundworms, hookworms and tapeworms, and flukes, which range in size from half an inch to many feet long. These parasites can cause diarrhea, constipation, weight loss, rectal itching, and, in the case of blood-eating hookworms, blood loss. Their eggs and larvae are generally spread in raw or improperly cooked pork or beef, contaminated vegetables or fruits, or the feces of infected individuals.

Good hygiene is one of the most important ways to avoid parasitical infection, because parasites are easily spread and may survive for very long periods outside a host. So wash your hands thoroughly before eating and after using the toilet, diapering your baby, pooper-scooping your dog, or cleaning your cat's litter box. Avoid going barefoot outside. Vacuum your house regularly. Wash all fruits and vegetables with soapy water, then rinse. Avoid raw meat and fish. Avoid water or ice from unfiltered sources. While these common-sense methods cannot completely protect you from parasites, they will greatly reduce your chances of getting infected by one.

The possibility of parasites must be considered when assessing the cause of your IBS. A parasite infection can usually be diagnosed by proper stool testing, and is usually readily treatable.

Renee

Renee had enjoyed good health her entire life, until suddenly, at the age of 30, she began suffering from poor digestion, fatigue, and intermittent diarrhea. She lost 15 pounds in one month, even though she was eating normally, and people began telling her she looked pale. "I could see it myself," said Renee. "My skin was almost green — not very attractive!"

Testing for food allergies proved negative. Stool testing, however, showed the presence of Giardia, *a parasite, in her stool. The doctor explained to Renee that the* Giardia *was affecting her ability to absorb carbohydrates, which explained her symptoms. Luckily, the doctor was able to prescribe an antiparasitic drug to kill the* Giardia, *and Renee rapidly regained her health.*

In response to the doctor's questions, Renee tried to pinpoint the source of her infection. She hadn't been swimming in any lakes or other natural water bodies, and she hadn't been drinking unfiltered water, nor had she purchased any fruits or vegetables from anywhere but the supermarket. Besides, she always washed them before she ate them.

It seemed like it would remain a mystery until Renee told her sister, who lived in another state, about her parasite infection. "Giardia!" exclaimed her sister. "But that's what Johnny had!" Johnny was Renee's 18-month-old nephew. "He picked it up at daycare," said Renee's sister. "It gave him and a bunch of other kids diarrhea, too."

But how could the Giardia *have traveled across state lines from Johnny to Renee? They hadn't visited each other in months. The only physical contact they had was when Renee's sister had sent a batch of homemade Christmas candy as a present. Could it be, Renee wondered, that her sister had changed Johnny's diapers and then went back to making candy, forgetting to wash her hands?*

Renee never found out the source of her Giardia *infection. But she never again ate her sister's Christmas food packages!*

Good guys to the rescue

Dysbiosis, or the presence of unwanted bacteria, yeast, or parasites in your intestines can be treated with a variety of pharmaceutical and/or botanical agents. Proper testing will generally determine exactly which agent is most effective.

A vital addition to your treatment, and one that is often overlooked by most doctors, is the replenishment of your intestinal tract with good bacteria. Remember, the antibiotic that kills the bad guys also kills the good ones. Therefore your treatment must include the use of supplements with friendly organisms such as *Lactobacillus acidophilus* and *Bifidobacterium*. Such supplements are called probiotics. They contain live bacteria which will greatly enhance your internal ecological system.

Taking high-quality probiotic supplements helps to ensure that there are enough good guys in your system to chase away the bad guys and prevent them from taking over territory. Unfortunately, the products available on the market vary widely in quality, and therefore in effectiveness. Good bacteria are

difficult to keep alive, and many products have little — if any
— living, or viable, bacteria left in them by the time you bring
them home.

Yogurt and acidophilus milk also contain good bacteria,
but you are unlikely to get enough good bacteria to correct an
imbalance just from eating yogurt or drinking acidophilus
milk. (In fact, if you have a dairy allergy then this is the
absolutely wrong thing to do.) You need the right strains of
bacteria, in high enough doses and still viable, in order to
experience the benefits of probiotics. An excellent source for
high quality probiotics is **www.qualityprobiotics.com**. This
issue is discussed further in Chapter 9.

Adding the right strains of friendly bacteria can have
dramatic medical benefits.   Although this concept has
been around for many years, more benefits continue to be
discovered through scientific studies.

Testing and treatment for bacteria, yeast, and parasites is
difficult and complex. It will be covered in the next chapter.

Content the stomach and
the stomach will content you.

Thomas Walker, English magistrate and writer
(1784 – 1836)

CHAPTER EIGHT

Stop Guessing!

Find out what's *really* wrong with you

Because IBS has been conventionally defined not by what it is, but by what it is not, successfully discovering its cause has been like trying to capture smoke in your hands. And treating IBS has been a constantly moving target – every time a new product or drug comes out you or your doctor gives it a try. It's really nothing more than a guessing game, and you get to be the guinea pig.

But now we *can* define it. As the previous chapters have shown, IBS symptoms are almost always caused by either food allergies, bacterial dysbiosis, yeast, or parasites. However, even saying that doesn't give you a firm target to treat unless you know which one (or more) is causing your IBS, and more specifically, exactly which food, bacteria, or parasite is the culprit.

Luckily we can determine this too. That's where testing comes in. Two kinds of tests are recommended: tests for food allergies, which are performed on your blood, and tests for bacteria, yeast, and parasites, which are done by stool testing.

Because most IBS sufferers have had their condition for months or even years, they may have both food allergies and bacterial dysbiosis going on. Their IBS may have started with a food allergy, but they may have taken antibiotics for it or for something else, even many years ago. The antibiotics killed off some bad bacteria, but snuffed out the good bacteria, too. This allowed unfriendly bacteria to move in and colonize, or yeast to take over the vacated space. Or they may have never had much good bacteria to begin with, and have never developed strong populations of good bacteria.

Blood and stool tests provide an easy way to sort this out. These tests are available, reasonably straightforward, and affordable, especially when you consider the benefit of having better health for the rest of your life. There is no need to continue wondering, guessing what is wrong and blindly spending money trying to find something that will help you.

You can *know*. And then you can do something that will end your IBS for good.

Matthew

Matthew is a rambunctious 5-year-old with a mischievous grin and the secret to perpetual motion. Even when he was feverish, which was often, Matthew didn't want to sit still.

Ever since he was a toddler Matthew had suffered from chronic ear infections. The pharmacists got to know Matthew's parents personally and joked that they kept a gallon jar full of Ampicillin handy, just for Matthew. He had been to the hospital to have tubes put in his ears to drain away the fluid that had accumulated behind his eardrums, caused by inflammation that never seemed to get completely better.

Even during the rare times when he didn't have an ear infection, Matthew suffered from insomnia. He woke up every two to three hours each night, complaining about stomachaches. It was difficult to get him to go back to sleep. Matthew's parents took turns getting up with Matthew, so they could each get some rest. Although they tried to maintain positive attitudes, it was hard. They grew irritable and fatigue was their daily companion. "When will he grow out of this?" they wondered in desperation.

Finally a blood allergy test was run on Matthew, and it showed elevated antibodies to dairy, eggs, strawberries, and sesame. Matthew's mother, delighted to find that there was a reason and a cure for Matthew's problems, totally revamped her kitchen and her cooking habits. She bought cookbooks on how to cook without dairy. She read every word on the labels of the food she bought.

Six months after being tested Matthew is still free from ear infections. He has also grown nearly three inches, and, best of all, he sleeps through the whole night — and so do his parents.

Food allergy testing

Food allergy testing is a highly specialized procedure performed only by doctors trained in recognizing and treating food allergies, and only in laboratories especially equipped to handle the sophisticated testing required. In order to give you an accurate result, this testing must be a blood test, and must include both IgE and IgG antibodies. If it does not evaluate both antibodies, there is a good possibility that the testing will miss your food allergy.

As noted in Chapter 6, skin testing is usually inadequate for diagnosing food allergies, and even the laboratories that do perform ELISA IgE and IgG blood testing are not all created equal. Food allergy testing is cutting-edge work. Many labs that claim to offer this testing have very poor quality control standards. Just because you have had IgE and IgG antibodies evaluated in the past does not guarantee that the lab work was properly performed. You should have your tests done by a lab which is a member of the College of American Pathologists. Such labs are required to undergo periodic comprehensive blinded testing. In addition, the lab should be certified and accredited under the Commission of Laboratory Accreditation. It also should perform daily in-house blinded split-sample reproducibility checks, using both positive and negative controls, in accordance with Clinical Laboratory Improvement Amendment proficiency testing criteria. The IBS Treatment Center works only with the very best laboratories in the country and tests them for consistently reliable and accurate results.

For you the procedure is neither complex nor difficult, and it is relatively painless. A blood sample will simply be drawn and sent to the lab. You are not required to fast, or to change your diet in any way, prior to blood collection. In fact, it is recommended that you not do so. (However, steroidal anti-inflammatory medications such as prednisone and corticosteroids may affect the results, so talk to your medical practitioner about these medications prior to testing.)

When the lab receives your blood, it performs the ELISA food allergy panel. The antibodies that your immune system creates against any of the foods in the panel are detected and measured. This test measures reactions to approximately 100 common foods, including dairy, beef, eggs, corn, soy, almonds, peanuts, wheat, seafood, and many others. (For a complete list, see Appendix B.)

Shelley

At 58, Shelley thought she should be used to constipation, since she'd had it for as long as she could remember. She had one to two bowel movements per week, and for the last ten years she had depended on laxatives to have even those. The stools she passed were small, hard, and round, more like rodent droppings. Abdominal cramps tormented her, often at night, which disrupted her sleep and that of her husband. Her husband began sleeping in a different bedroom so he could get some sleep. Shelley didn't blame him, but she felt lonely and deserted.

In addition, Shelley had recently been diagnosed with high blood pressure and given a prescription for Atenolol. This medication seemed to make her constipation even worse.

Then Shelley began to suffer from searing heartburn as well. A friend who had previously suffered from heartburn told Shelley about the blood allergy testing she had done, which had shown her which foods were causing the heartburn. "What have I got to lose?" thought Shelley.

Shelley's tests showed a high allergy to eggs and plums. After removing these two items from her diet, not only did Shelley's heartburn disappear, but so did her constipation. She began having one bowel movement a day, without the aid of laxatives — to her a marvelous thing. Her blood pressure dropped to normal and she was able to discontinue her medication. And best of all, her husband moved back into the bedroom.

ELISA stands for Enzyme Linked Immunosorbent Assay, which describes the biochemical process whereby antibodies are detected in your blood. As mentioned in Chapter 6, this test directly measures your immune system's response to food, and what you eat on the day of the test does not affect the results. A standard ELISA food allergy panel will measure both IgG and IgE antibodies, unlike other food allergy testing. It sounds complex, but the ELISA test is relatively simple to explain.

ELISA is a semi-quantitative test, meaning that it can measure the amount of antibodies in your blood. It works like this: Your blood is drawn, put into a tube, set aside to clot, and then spun in a centrifuge, which separates the portion containing the antibodies. This portion is then removed from the tube and sent to the lab for evaluation, where it is added to a plate made up of small wells, each of which has been coated with a small amount of a single purified food protein. If your blood contains any antibodies to one of the foods, they will bind with that food. The amount of binding indicates the number of antibodies being produced by your immune system. The more antibodies, the stronger your immune system is reacting to the food. The findings are then summarized for you in an easy-to-understand report and bar graph.

If you have no food allergies, no antibodies will be detected. However, when IBS sufferers are tested, a very high percentage of them have antibodies to one or more foods. When they stop eating those foods and are treated for any deficiencies related to the allergy, they invariably feel better.

In addition to the ELISA panel, a blood test for celiac disease should also be run. As discussed in Chapter 6, celiac disease is a special form of gluten/wheat intolerance. Although gluten and wheat are included in the ELISA food panel, celiac disease cannot be ruled out based on the results of the ELISA panel alone. This highly specialized diagnosis can be ruled out only after you have been tested for tissue transglutaminase antibodies and total IgA.

The ELISA Standard Food Allergy Panel is the most accurate method known for determining food allergies. It is much more effective than skin testing. This test takes the guesswork out of treating your IBS, and saves you a great deal of time, effort, and discomfort. And if by chance your ELISA panel happens to be negative, you can quickly move on to other potential causes of your problem without spending valuable time on an unsuccessful elimination diet and then wondering if you actually did it correctly.

After your Standard Food Allergy Panel is completed, the results will be sent to your physician. See Appendix C for an example of what your results will look like. Unless you are medically trained in recognizing food allergies, you must consult with your physician to fully understand your test results. As the television ads say, do not try this at home!

The IBS Treatment Center provides you with both comprehensive, detailed counseling to help you evaluate your test results and extensive recommendations for treatment. This is covered in the next chapter.

Jerry

Six months ago 27-year-old Jerry seemed at the peak of health and fitness. He had been a "jock" throughout high school and college, and maintained his athletic prowess as he got older. He was the star player on the community softball team, he skied like a pro, he lifted weights, and he ran marathons. He was proud of his athletic ability and his muscled, toned body.

Then Jerry began suffering from a host of digestive and other complaints. He had loose stools and excessive gas. He lost a lot of weight and, no matter what he did, couldn't seem to gain it back. He developed severe acne on his back. He was always tired, and his endurance plummeted so much that just running around the track at the gym tired him out.

His doctor suggested he be tested for allergies. Jerry hooted at the idea. "I'm not allergic," he stated positively. "I've always been able to eat anything!" His doctor explained that although he may have been allergic all his life, the symptoms may have been hiding until now. So Jerry agreed to the blood tests, although he was sure it was a waste of time.

Jerry was still suspicious when the allergy testing revealed a severe allergy to gluten. "Nah, that can't be," he scoffed. But he agreed to remove all gluten products from his diet, just to see what would happen. He had to eat his words when his IBS symptoms cleared up completely within two days. In two weeks, the acne on his back was gone. And in two months Jerry was back in training for his next marathon.

Bacteria, yeast, and parasite testing

If your Standard Food Allergy Panel comes back negative for food allergies, it is highly probable that the answer to your IBS will show up on the Comprehensive Stool Bacteria, Yeast, and Parasite Analysis. This test shows the amount of friendly bacteria, unfriendly bacteria, and yeast growing in your digestive tract. If requested, it can also include an evaluation for parasites, including the most common ones such as *Giardia, Cryptosporidium, Blastocystis hominis,* tapeworms, and hookworms. The Comprehensive Stool Bacteria, Yeast, and Parasite Analysis is different from standard stool tests, which evaluate only parasites or the ugly bacteria that cause potentially life-threatening bloody diarrhea. Standard tests do not cover the wealth of other bacteria, yeast, and parasites whose presence or absence can lead to IBS.

As in testing for food allergies, your part in the process is simple. Simpler, in fact, because after you visit the clinic, you can gather stool samples in the privacy and comfort of your own home. You then send this sample directly to the lab for testing.

The lab's part is considerably more complex, and some labs do a much better job than others at this kind of specialized testing. It is wise to trust your medical practitioner when selecting a lab.

The stool sample is examined under a microscope to check for the presence of yeast and parasites. To test for bacteria and yeast, a culture is grown in a petri dish. In order for the culture to grow, the bacteria and yeast must be fed; otherwise they will just die. Since different bacteria and yeast eat different things, the nutrients fed to them must be selectively applied.

Once the lab has identified a certain bacteria or yeast, they will try to kill it with a variety of different antibacterial or antifungal agents, both pharmaceutical and natural. This is called sensitivity and resistance testing, and it enables the lab to recommend the treatment appropriate for each patient. For example, the most common treatment for *Candida* is the drug Nystatin, which is usually very safe and effective. But the lab may discover that your particular strain of *Candida* is resistant to Nystatin, and note this on your test results. Therefore another drug will be suggested and will need to be selected.

Because parasites can be difficult to detect, testing for them may be even more complicated. Parasites are often detectable only by their eggs or cysts, which are not shed consistently from one day to the next. Therefore most labs will request that stool samples be collected on three consecutive days. Evaluating specimens over several days greatly increases the detection rate for parasites.

When your tests are complete, the results and recommendations for treatment will be sent to your physician, who will then need to spend the time necessary to explain these tests to you. Appendix D shows you what the report may look like, but be aware that you must have a qualified physician help you understand and evaluate your options for treatment. Some of these options will be discussed in the next chapter.

*Happiness: a good bank account,
a good cook, and a good digestion.*

**Jean-Jacques Rousseau,
French philosopher and writer
(1712 – 1778)**

CHAPTER NINE

Free at Last

Once the lab work is in

If you are like the majority of IBS sufferers, you are delighted and relieved to know that your IBS has an identifiable cause. Now you'd like to know the solution, right?

Good news: there is a solution for you. Whether your IBS is caused by a food allergy, a bacterial imbalance, a parasite, or a combination of the three, once the tests have been run and the cause identified, it can be addressed. But like the condition itself, the treatment and cure for your IBS will be uniquely yours. No single answer fits all. In fact, you can waste a lot of time, energy, and money trying generic solutions that work for some people, but which are totally inappropriate for you.

Treatment plans for food allergies

Once the offending foods have been discovered, the next step is to eliminate them from your diet. Sounds easy, doesn't it? As has been shown, it isn't always so. But it doesn't have to be difficult, and it can even be fun — especially when you start to feel so much better.

You will learn a great deal about the make-up of your foods, and how to nourish yourself in a healthy way. Education is necessary to make sure that you can identify all sources of the offending foods. Learning how to identify the foods that are causing the problem and where to find the foods that you *can* eat is essential to the long-term resolution of your IBS.

It is usually recommended that you eliminate all the foods to which your body reacts — the "cold turkey" approach– for at least 6 weeks. This is the surest and quickest route to curing your problem. However, you don't need to feel deprived; there are many nutritious and delicious substitutes available for nearly every food. (And many other not so nutritious options too!) Many people have discovered "new" (to them) foods that quickly become their favorites. Look on it as an adventure in eating.

Some people make a game out of finding the hidden sources for their reactive foods. In order to experience the highest level of improvement possible, you must learn to read and understand the labels on the foods you buy. If someone else does the shopping in your house, he or she too must be educated on reading labels and in knowing what to look for. Be especially careful of packaged foods that are rich in preservatives and artificial flavorings, sweeteners, and colorings, often hidden sources of reactive foods. You should go through your kitchen cupboards and read the labels on everything there — then throw out the offenders or give them to your local food bank.

You, or whoever cooks in your house, will learn to cook with different ingredients. You probably won't have to give up your favorite "comfort foods" — you'll just learn to make them in a new, healthier way. Many cookbooks on the market can help you adapt and will give you lots of ideas for healthy, creative dishes.

When dining out, you'll learn that you can be assertive in choosing restaurants and menu selections. You'll also learn that good service includes being able to describe how foods are prepared so that customers can avoid food allergens. A good idea is to dine at restaurants with a large variety of selections so you have many choices. And occasionally you will be the envy of your friends when a chef actually takes a personal interest in preparing a special meal just for you. Depending on your food allergy and location, you may even find some restaurants that cater to folks like you!

At the IBS Treatment Center, each client meets one-on-one with a physician to discuss his or her lab results in great detail, so that they are thoroughly understood. Each client is also given a wealth of supportive information specifically related to his or her food allergy. This includes pamphlets on hidden sources of reactive foods; education in reading labels; shopping resources; recommendations for cookbooks and restaurants; product recommendations; and referrals to nutritionists who are experts in creating healthy, nutritious diets for people with food allergies.

Lucy

Lucy and her husband Jack were in their early thirties and had been trying to get pregnant for more than three years. They were starting to get desperate and wondering if they would ever have a family.

Lucy had always had an abnormally long menstrual cycle of 35 days. She also suffered from gas, bloating, edema, and chronic fatigue. She often had dark circles under her eyes. During her periods those circles seemed even darker to Lucy — in fact, everything seemed dark on the days her periods started.

Lucy and Jack underwent the standard fertility tests and all the results were normal. There should have been no reason why they couldn't conceive. Yet they didn't.

Lucy consulted the IBS Treatment Center about her symptoms of gas and bloating. She didn't mention her infertility because she did not connect the two problems. The physician suggested testing for a food allergy. Sure enough, Lucy's results showed positive for gluten, dairy, corn, and garlic.

Lucy was delighted when the removal of the allergens from her diet eliminated her gas and bloating. She was pleasantly surprised to find that she had more energy and the dark circles under her eyes disappeared. An even bigger surprise was that her next period came 28 days after the last one, instead of 35.

And she was absolutely astounded when four months later she became pregnant.

Treatment plans for bacterial imbalances, yeast, and parasites

If your test results show that you have insufficient good bacteria or that inappropriate bacteria, yeast, or parasites are present, it is just as important to treat these conditions as it is to treat food allergies. They alone can cause IBS, or they can contribute to the effects of a food allergy. In particular, a deficiency of good bacteria is associated with a higher incidence of many symptoms of food allergies, especially in children. Bacterial or fungal imbalances are readily treatable, as are parasites, and once corrected will result in tremendous improvement in your health.

Treating bad bacteria

The lab results from the stool tests include information not only on which, if any, unfriendly bacteria, yeast, or parasites are present in your system, but also on which agents, pharmaceutical and natural, are the most likely to destroy them. There are many strains of the same bacteria; the *Citrobacter*, for example, in your system may be sensitive to tetracycline (a pharmaceutical agent), while the *Citrobacter* in someone else's digestive tract may be markedly resistant to the same drug. If your lab results show that your *Pseudomonas* is resistant to Uva Ursi (a botanical antibiotic), it will do no good at all to take it, even if it worked wonders for your grandmother. This is why is it critical to have a qualified physician work with you to determine the best way to rid yourself of bad bacteria, yeast, or parasites.

Probiotics: Adding the good bacteria

Just as important as destroying the bad guys, and just as often overlooked in the medical world, is the reseeding of your digestive tract with good bacteria, or probiotics. Regardless of which agent is used to destroy the bad guys, you must assume that it is having a negative effect on the good guys, too. This is true even if a natural or botanical agent is used. If the bad guys are dying, so are the good guys.

A deficiency of good bacteria is problematic even if there are no bad bacteria present. Replenishing the digestive tract with probiotics encourages a healthier intestinal ecosystem. Probiotic foods and supplements contain live friendly bacteria, such as *Lactobacilli acidophilus* and *Bifidobacterium*. Remember, you cannot have enough of these good bacteria. Their presence inhibits the growth of bad bacteria and yeast and is your best protection against becoming reinfected.

Many people take acidophilus in a product from their neighborhood grocery store or health-food store, and think they have done enough. This is not necessarily true! Although there are dozens of supplement products marketed as probiotics, they are not equally effective.

First, many products do not contain enough bacteria to correct a deficiency. Remember, the bacteria in your system number around 100 trillion. When reseeding, you must add enough good bacteria to colonize territory and discourage the unhealthy bacteria from moving in again. For instance, a fairly good probiotic product might have around 4 billion organisms per capsule, which sounds like a lot. But that is still well under one-tenth of 1% of the total number of bacteria in your intestinal tract. And many products contain far fewer than 4 billion organisms. You may need to take an especially high potency probiotic product, which can have from 100 to 200 billion organisms per packet (usually taken in water), for several days to build up your colonies of healthy bacteria.

Another significant problem with probiotic products is quality control. Many products contain little, if any, living bacteria. Probiotics are very difficult to keep alive. The products must be either constantly refrigerated or freeze-dried for the probiotics to remain viable. Even if they are freeze-dried, they should be refrigerated until sold in order to maintain their viability. If stored improperly, they will do you little good.

Lactobacillus acidophilus and *Bifidobacterium*, the two most important probiotics, come in a variety of strains. These strains vary in their effectiveness in treating IBS. Better strains survive better at the pH of the digestive tract, adhere better to the lining of the intestine, and are more effective at curing IBS.

Prebiotics are nearly as important as probiotics, for without them the friendly bacteria will die. Prebiotics are foods or supplements that contain nutrients required by these bacteria to grow and thrive. The best-known prebiotics are fructooligosaccharides (FOS), which can be found naturally in foods such as onions, leeks, garlic, and artichokes, as well as in other vegetables and some grains. They are also available in supplement form.

FOS are molecular chains made up of the sugar fructose. The size and complexity of the FOS chain is what makes it beneficial, because the body does not quickly absorb FOS as it does the simple sugar fructose. FOS do tend to have a sweet taste, but they do not affect blood sugar levels. Because the body does not have the ability to ferment or breakdown FOS, they act more like a fiber than a sugar. Beneficial bacteria, however, can ferment FOS and use them as food. This process also results in the production of short chain fatty acids, which provide nutrition for the cells of the intestinal lining. Therefore, FOS promote the growth of friendly bacteria, directly resulting in a healthier digestive tract.

You should be forewarned that taking a high potency probiotic product may temporarily cause gas, bloating, and some discomfort. This perfectly normal reaction is caused by a change in how your foods are being fermented by bacteria and means that positive changes are taking place in the bacterial environment of your intestines. You must continue treatment at least until the gas subsides, or you will not have replaced all of the unwanted bacteria. This may take up to a week or more. It's a little bit like exercising. If you haven't worked out for a while, your muscles hurt when you start exercising again. If you give up and stop, you never get in shape. But if you keep on training, you get beyond the aches and become stronger.

Due to the importance of probiotics and prebiotics and to the wide disparity in product quality, the IBS Treatment Center critically evaluates these products and offers only the very best ones. See **www.qualityprobiotics.com** or **www.bestbacteria.com** for high-quality probiotics and for further information on this subject.

The IBS Treatment Center

The IBS Treatment Center is dedicated solely to the diagnosis and treatment of IBS. Although located in Seattle, Washington, the IBS Treatment Center treats people from all over the United States and Canada. Because we are totally focused on this particular condition, our goal is to be the best possible source of care, treatment, education, and advice for anyone seeking help with their IBS.

The IBS Treatment Center offers the potential for curing IBS where none had existed before. Unlike most other health care options for IBS, we get to the cause of the problem, putting an end to the symptoms without the long-term use of medications, supplements, or digestive aids. We spend the time getting to know you and your problem so that we can determine exactly how to cure it. You are not treated like a statistic. You are given the personal attention required to get to the help that you need.

Your first office visit at the IBS Treatment Center is a long face-to-face meeting with the physician, often taking thirty minutes or more. Return visits are also long, in order to allow enough time for the physician to educate you about your condition and the required treatment. These extended visits, which are longer than typical appointments with a doctor, allow us to truly understand you and to properly assess your needs and problems. A strong relationship based on good communication is key to the success of the program, and this kind of relationship is not built in five or ten minutes spent with a harassed doctor trying to see as many patients as possible.

At the IBS Treatment Center your concerns are truly heard, you are treated with respect, and your questions are honestly answered. The extra time also allows you to receive the information you need to attain the highest level of success possible in your treatment program. All treatment recommendations, which are customized to your specific needs, are thoroughly discussed, and a written copy of the treatment plan, recommendations, resources, and other assistance is provided for you to take home.

In addition to the treatment of current conditions, the IBS Treatment Center focuses on the prevention of future health problems. We work with you as part of a team effort to create a treatment plan that is both effective and "do-able." Again, education is a cornerstone of the effectiveness of this aspect of our program.

After your initial consultation, the IBS Treatment Center can provide follow-up over the telephone, to accommodate those clients who live outside the Seattle area.

The critical point to remember is that interpreting your lab results and creating an effective treatment plan can be a relatively involved endeavor. To succeed at eliminating your IBS, it is crucial that you receive expert guidance from your health care provider.

Carol

Carol was 41 and had never really known what it was like to feel "normal." She had a lifetime history of nausea, vomiting, and constipation alternating with loose stools. As a baby she was colicky and spat up constantly. As a toddler she had ear infection after ear infection, requiring antibiotics and the insertion of tubes in her ears. In high school, she had chronic sinus infections. When she became an adult, fatigue plagued her. Her libido was low, even though she was married to a man she loved.

The many doctors whom Carol had seen, including gastroenterologists, had not been able to find anything wrong with her physically. Most suggested that anxiety was the cause of her problems. Carol's mother agreed with them. "Carol's a bundle of nerves," she told everyone. She seemed to be proud of it.

It's true that Carol suffered from anxiety. So many years of sickness will do that to a person. She worried not only that she would die young, but also that it would be her own fault. "They'll write, 'It was all in her head' on my tombstone," she joked morbidly.

When it was suggested to Carol that food allergies could be the cause of her problem, she laughed scornfully. "That would be way too easy," she scoffed. "The doctors never told me I had allergies." But urged by her husband, Carol agreed to have blood tests.

The tests showed a strong allergy to dairy and eggs. Carol was dumfounded, and at first, unbelieving. But when she removed all dairy and egg products from her diet, her health improved dramatically. For the first time in her life, Carol went an entire week without throwing up. Her stools were completely normal — no constipation, no diarrhea. In two weeks, she felt strong and full of energy. Instead of listlessly agreeing to sex, Carol herself initiated sex with her husband (who was delighted). And the best part of all was that Carol's anxiety seemed to have melted away. Now her life seems full of promise.

Life without IBS

Whether your IBS was caused by a food allergy, bacterial imbalance, parasites, or a combination of all three, with proper treatment it can become a thing of the past. And with the proper education you can make sure it *stays* in the past.

All those who told you there was no cure for IBS were wrong. There is a cause, a cure, and an effective treatment for IBS.

The world is round, and the
place which may seem like the end
may actually be the beginning.

Ivy Baker Priest,
U.S. Treasurer, (1905 – 1975)

CHAPTER TEN

Feeling Good

The rest of the story

Remember Jennifer, Carl, and Linda, whose stories began this book? They are fictional characters, but stories like theirs really happen, every day. And the best thing about these stories is that they have happy endings.

Jennifer

There was still a month to go before the Junior Prom when Jennifer visited the IBS Treatment Center for the first time. "This was like my last chance," said Jennifer in her usual dramatic fashion. "I had tried everything, but then I heard that this place could cure IBS, so I asked my mom if I could go there. I mean, what did I have to lose?"

After hearing that Jennifer's symptoms were gas and constipation alternating with diarrhea, the doctor recommended she be tested for food allergies by means of the simple blood test. "I was pretty surprised," said Jennifer. "My friend Gayle has food allergies — she swells up like a balloon if she even looks at a strawberry — and I thought all food allergies were like that. I never knew they could make you constipated."

When Jennifer's results came back from the lab, she went to the IBS Treatment Center to see the doctor. They went over the chart together.

"The chart was pretty easy to read," Jennifer said. "The doctor explained the difference between the IgG and IgE reactions. I didn't have any IgE reactions, which are the kind Gayle probably has to strawberries. But my IgG reactions — wow! Some of them were like really high!"

Jennifer's chart showed high IgG reactions to all forms of dairy and moderate reactions to bananas and broccoli. "They told me I might be able to eat bananas and broccoli in moderation," said Jennifer, "although I didn't really care. I mean, I like bananas, but I can live without them. And I loathe broccoli, so I was sort of glad I was allergic to it, since now I never have to eat it again.

"But the dairy thing, that was hard. I mean, I was reactive to *all* dairy foods — cow's milk, all kinds of cheese, yogurt, ice cream, butter, you name it. If it comes from a cow, my body just doesn't like it."

Jennifer, along with her mother, climbed a steep learning curve over the next few weeks. "I had no idea how much I used milk, butter, and cheese in my everyday cooking," said Jennifer's mom. "I put milk and butter in the mashed potatoes, I put cheese on every pasta dish I made, I sprinkled parmesan on salads. I had to break the habit and learn how to cook without dairy, or to find substitutes."

"Yeah, like macaroni and cheese," chimed in Jennifer. "It's my favorite food in the whole world, practically since I was a baby, and my mom made it *soo* good. I was really bummed because I thought I would have to give it up. But Mom went on a hunt for a good recipe using soy cheese, and after a few weird tries, she found one. I was very happy that I didn't have to give it up after all."

Jennifer learned to change the way she ate out, too. She and her friends liked to hang out at a local pizza place after school, eating pizza and gossiping about the latest school news. Sometimes they went to a nearby espresso bar and splurged on lattes and scones. "It took me a while to find something I could eat *and* like," said Jennifer. "I like herbal teas, so it wasn't too hard at the espresso bar, although I couldn't eat scones or muffins, because most baked goods are made with whey. But it was pretty funny trying to convince the pizza place to make me a small pizza without cheese. They looked at me like I was crazy or something. But you know what? They got used to it. When I'd come in, the people behind the counter go, 'Hey, here comes the no-cheese girl!'"

The most difficult lesson for Jennifer and her family was that dairy pops up in places they didn't expect. It was not enough to remove the more obvious dairy foods like milk, cheese, and butter. They learned that lactalbumin, casein, and whey, all milk-derived proteins or by-products, are present in a vast array of foods, especially packaged and processed foods. "There were at least three pages in the booklet I was given," said Jennifer, "just listing the hidden sources of dairy. I was blown away when I found out that margarine, muffins, canned and packaged soups, sausages, and sherbet all contain casein. So does caramel color and caramel flavoring, and if you read the labels on stuff, that's added to a bunch of foods to preserve them or improve their flavor. And I can't eat casein."

Instead of becoming frustrated, Jennifer made a game out of searching for the hidden dairy in foods. "It was kind of like those silly kid's games where you find the seven Abraham Lincolns hidden in one picture," she laughed. "Only I was looking for the hidden cows! It didn't take long before I was pretty good at it, too."

By the time the prom rolled around, Jennifer felt better than she had in years. Her eyes were bright and her smile lit up the room. Her alternating diarrhea and constipation had gone away. The new dress she had bought fit snug around her abdomen, but she wasn't worried. She was no longer suffering from bloating, gas, or abdominal pain.

At the fancy restaurant where she and Tom had dinner before the prom, Jennifer ordered salmon and asked the waiter to make sure it was cooked without butter, explaining she was allergic to dairy. ("Deathly allergic" was how she put it, typically dramatic, although she was laughing as she spoke.) She had a salad with walnuts and balsamic vinegar dressing. Instead of a baked potato with butter and sour cream she ordered asparagus. "Remember, no butter!" she told the waiter. "You wouldn't want me to *explode*, would you? It would really mess up your dining room!" They all laughed.

"So yeah, there are some things I can't eat," said Jennifer recently. "But so what? It's such a small — such a *tiny* — price to pay for feeling good every day. For not having to run to the bathroom six or seven times a day. For not being afraid I'm going to embarrass myself in front of my friends. For living like a normal person, having fun instead of worry and pain. Gosh, what's a little cheese compared to all that?"

Carl

"IBS is a good name for it," said Carl sourly at his first visit to the IBS Treatment Center. "I think IBS really stands for 'It's B.S.'"

Carl was often grouchy. He came to the IBS Treatment Center after his wife heard about it and pressured him to go. He finally agreed, although he was reluctant. "I bet they won't be able to do anything either," he told her.

Carl told the doctor about his symptom of recurring diarrhea. When the doctor probed into Carl's history and found out that the IBS began after Carl's knee surgery, he suggested that antibiotics might have caused Carl's system to become unbalanced.

Carl disagreed. "Nope, that can't be it," he declared, "because my wife read about that on some medical site on the Internet, and she bought some acidophilus like it recommended. I've been taking it for months and nothing has changed."

The doctor smiled and commented mildly, "Well, there's acidophilus and there's acidophilus. Why don't we start by doing some tests to see if there is an imbalance or not?"

Carl agreed, although he was less than delighted about the process. "It was pretty gross," he said, "like pooper-scooping after yourself, instead of your dog." But he gathered a sample and sent it off to the lab.

Sure enough, Carl's lab results showed that his system lacked good bacteria and had too much of the unfriendly kind. The doctor explained Carl's results to him.

"You're supposed to have beneficial flora, the good guys, in high amounts, but I had zero," said Carl. "No *Bifidobacterium*, no *Lactobacillus*. That was a problem all by itself, but I had an even bigger one — I had a 4+ of *Pseudomanus aeruginosa*, a nasty little bacteria that I probably picked up in the hospital.

"What a relief it was to see those results," said Carl, smiling. "I felt vindicated, because every time I had been told there was nothing wrong with me, I *knew* there was. And those tests proved it."

The first step in Carl's healing was to kill the *Pseudomanus aeruginosa*. The lab showed that this particular strain was sensitive to the antibiotic Cipro, and the doctor gave Carl a prescription. Carl took the Cipro for two weeks, and started to feel better within a few days. His diarrhea cleared up, never to return.

After Carl finished the Cipro, he was given a course of high-quality probiotics to reseed his intestinal tract. Carl called it "bug building," and took his daily capsules as diligently as he worked out at the gym.

It took a few months for Carl's system to get completely back to normal, and while his bug building was going on, he suffered from bloating and gas, which his doctor explained was normal. "It was no big deal," remarked Carl.

Three months after Carl came to the IBS Treatment Center, his health was fully restored. No more diarrhea, no more gas. He and his wife took a vacation and revisited Hawaii. This time Carl joined his wife in scuba diving.

"Bad bugs!" says Carl now, laughing heartily. "That's all it was — the wrong kind of bugs were bugging me! Now I love my bugs and they love me."

Linda

"I think I'm going to quit my job," Linda said the first time she visited the IBS Treatment Center. "I just feel so awful all the time. I've had to call in substitute teachers three times in the last two months, and even when I am there I know I'm not doing a great job. It's not fair to the children." Her eyes filled with tears. "I used to love my job," she whispered. "But now most of the time I just don't care."

The doctor listened to Linda's long history of various complaints, including constipation and the severe abdominal pain that made it necessary for her to take Vicodin. Because Linda's symptoms were so varied and had persisted for so long, the doctor recommended that they test both her blood for possible food allergies and her stool for bacterial imbalance.

When her tests came back from the lab Linda and her doctor had a long conversation about the results, which showed that Linda indeed suffered from the "double whammy" of allergies and unfriendly bacteria.

"My IgG reactions were off the scale for eggs, both whites and yolks," she said, "and were also very high for coconut. I had moderate reactions to sesame and mushrooms. When I first read those results, I thought they didn't make much sense, because although I like eggs, I don't eat them every day. And I hardly ever eat coconut. So why did I have such severe symptoms?"

Then Linda began learning about the hidden sources of her particular reactive foods. "I couldn't believe how many foods have eggs added to them," she said. "Like most baked goods such as muffins, cookies, and cakes; ice cream; breakfast cereals; marshmallows; mayonnaise; bologna; sausages, even tartar sauce!

"And processed or packaged foods often have dried or powdered eggs added to them as binders," she added. "I had to read every label and look for words like *albumin* and *globulin*, and any ingredient beginning with the prefix *ovo*, which is Latin for *egg*."

Coconut was an even bigger surprise. "It's those processed foods again," she said, shaking her head in amazement. "Many of them, including bakery goods, contain coconut oil! But many labels don't *say* coconut oil — they say MCT oil (for medium chain triglycerides) or sodium laurel sulfate, which is used to improve consistency in some foods, and is a derivative of — guess — coconut!

"Now how is an average person supposed to know that?" she wondered. "It's no wonder I felt so awful all the time. Nearly every day on my way to work I would stop by the neighborhood espresso stand and buy a cup of coffee and a muffin for breakfast. Those muffins looked so innocent. Who would have guessed that to me they were poison?"

While Linda was learning how to eliminate the offending foods from her diet, she was also dealing with the bacterial imbalance her tests had shown. Her beneficial flora showed a 4+ for *Lactobacillus* and a 4+ for beneficial *E. coli*, but only a 1+ for *Bifidobacterium*, well under the optimum range. The tests also showed the presence of *Citrobacter freundii*. "I looked it up on the Internet," said Linda, "and it really is a bad little guy. I wanted it out of me right away. My tests showed that my particular strain was sensitive to a few natural agents, which pleased me. I didn't want to take any more drugs than I had to.

"Uva Ursi was one of the natural substances that the tests said would kill the *Citrobacter* in my system, so we started with that. Because I like to know about things, I read up on it. Uva Ursi is an evergreen shrub that is also called bearberry, because bears like to eat the berries in the spring. I used what I learned about Uva Ursi in a natural history lesson for my fifth graders. They were intrigued that I, like the bears, made use of this plant."

To Linda's delight, the Uva Ursi worked and killed the *Citrobacter freundii*. She was then given a course of probiotics to build up her colonies of friendly bacteria.

Within just a few months, Linda's life had changed dramatically. "I can't say I'm back to normal," she said, "because to me normal meant fatigue, sickness, and pain. And that's just what I don't have any more. I sleep through the night, my bowel movements are regular and easy, and best of all I have no more abdominal pain. I no longer take Vicodin!"

Linda didn't quit her job after all. Instead she rediscovered how much she loved teaching. The racket that a class full of 10-year-olds can make while learning didn't bother her; in fact she liked it. She said it sounded like music. At home, she laughed and joked around with her teenage children, who suddenly appeared to be quite nice people after all.

"The other night my husband and I went out to dinner and a movie," she said recently. "It sounds like such a little thing — just dinner and a movie. But to me it was a big deal, because I felt wonderful that whole evening. The food tasted great, my husband was charming, and we held hands all through the movie. The movie was a comedy, and even though it wasn't that funny, I found myself laughing out loud in the theater, just because it felt so good to really laugh."

The end of IBS

Jennifer, Carl, and Linda are laughing with joy. Their lives are theirs to enjoy, and they no longer spend them in discomfort, worry, or embarrassment.

If IBS has squelched the laughter in your life, take heart. Find out what causes your IBS. Do something about it. Laugh and have fun. Get on with your life.

APPENDICES

APPENDIX A

Symptoms Commonly Caused by Food Allergies

Foods are not the only cause of these conditions, but in a great number of cases they are the primary cause. Anyone who suffers from these should be screened for food allergies.

Abdominal pain
Acne
ADD
ADHD
Anal itching
Anaphylaxis
Anxiety
Arthritis
Asthma
Bad breath
Bed-wetting
Bloating
Canker sores
Chronic fatigue
Colic
Congestion
Constipation
Coughing, chronic
Dark circles under eyes
Depression
Dermatitis
Diarrhea
Dizziness
Dry skin

Ear infections
Eczema
Encopresis
Fatigue
Fibromyalgia
Flatulence
Flushing
Foggy mind
Frequent colds or flus
Gagging
Gas
Gastrointestinal bleeding
Hayfever
Headaches
Heartburn
Hives
Hoarseness
Hypoglycemia
Idiopathic thrombocytopenic purpura (ITP;
    low platelet count)
Indigestion
Insomnia
Iron deficiency anemia
Irritability
Irritable bowel syndrome (IBS)
Itchy skin
Itchy intestines
ITP (idiopathic thrombocytopenic purpura,
    low platelet count)
Joint pain
Juvenile rheumatoid arthritis
Meniere's disease
Mental fogginess
Migraines
Nausea

Osteoporosis
Osteopenia
Palpitations
Premenstrual syndrome
Poor growth
Poor immune function
Protein-losing enteropathy
Psoriasis
Reflux
Rheumatoid arthritis
Runny nose
Schizophrenia
Seizures
Sinusitis
Spitting up
Styes
Swelling of hands or feet
Urinary tract infections
Urticaria
Vaginal itching
Vitamin B_{12} deficiency
Vomiting
Weight gain
Weight loss

APPENDIX B

Foods Included in the Standard Food Allergy Panel

Dairy
Casein
Cheddar cheese
Cottage cheese
Milk, cow
Milk, goat
Mozzarella cheese
Whey
Yogurt

Grains
Amaranth
Barley
Buckwheat
Corn
Gliadin, wheat
Gluten, wheat
Oat
Rice, white
Rye
Spelt
Wheat, whole

Nuts
Almond
Coconut
Filbert
Peanut

Pecan
Sesame
Sunflower seed
Walnut

Legumes
Green pea
Kidney bean
Lentil
Lima bean
Peanut
Pinto bean
Soy bean
String bean

Meat and Fowl
Beef
Chicken
Egg white, chicken
Egg yolk, chicken
Lamb
Pork
Turkey

Seafood
American lobster
Atlantic cod
Dungeness crab
Halibut
Manila clam
Oyster
Pacific salmon
Red snapper
Sole
Western shrimp

Yellowfin tuna
Vegetables
Asparagus
Avacado
Beet
Bell pepper, green
Broccoli
Cabbage, white
Carrot
Cauliflower
Celery
Cucumber
Garlic
Green Squash
Lettuce
Mushroom, common
Olive, black
Onion, white
Potato, white
Pumpkin
Radish
Spinach, green
Sweet potato
Tomato, red
Zucchini squash

Fruits
Apple
Apricot
Banana
Blueberry
Cranberry
Grape, red
Grapefruit
Lemon

Orange
Papaya
Peach
Pear
Pineapple
Plum
Raspberry
Strawberry

Miscellaneous

Baker's yeast
Brewer's yeast
Cocoa bean (chocolate)
Coffee bean
Honey
Sugar cane

This list is subject to change without notice.

APPENDIX C

Sample Test Results from the Standard Food Allergy Panel

Note: The black bar represents IgE antibodies. The white bar represents IgG antibodies. An elevation in either antibody is significant. Notice the very high immune/antibody response to all dairy products and to chicken eggs in this sample patient.

(See next page)

Food Allergy Test Page 1

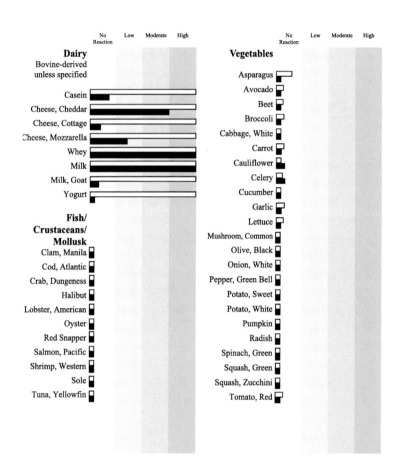

Food Allergy Test Page 2

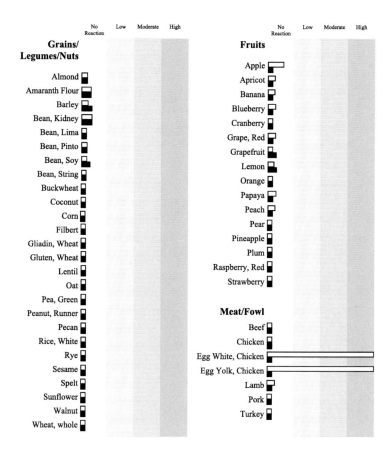

	No Reaction	Low	Moderate	High
Grains/ Legumes/Nuts				
Almond				
Amaranth Flour				
Barley				
Bean, Kidney				
Bean, Lima				
Bean, Pinto				
Bean, Soy				
Bean, String				
Buckwheat				
Coconut				
Corn				
Filbert				
Gliadin, Wheat				
Gluten, Wheat				
Lentil				
Oat				
Pea, Green				
Peanut, Runner				
Pecan				
Rice, White				
Rye				
Sesame				
Spelt				
Sunflower				
Walnut				
Wheat, whole				

	No Reaction	Low	Moderate	High
Fruits				
Apple				
Apricot				
Banana				
Blueberry				
Cranberry				
Grape, Red				
Grapefruit				
Lemon				
Orange				
Papaya				
Peach				
Pear				
Pineapple				
Plum				
Raspberry, Red				
Strawberry				
Meat/Fowl				
Beef				
Chicken				
Egg White, Chicken				
Egg Yolk, Chicken				
Lamb				
Pork				
Turkey				

A P P E N D I X D

Sample Test Results from Comprehensive Bacteria and Yeast Panel

MICROBIOLOGY

Bacteriology Culture		
Beneficial flora (bacteria)	Imbalances	Dysbiotic (bad) flora
Bifidobacter 0 Lactobacillus acidophilus 0		Pseudomonas aeruginosa 4+ Klebsiella 3+

Mycology (Yeast) Culture

Normal flora	Dysbiotic flora (bad)
	Candida albicans 3+

	Normal	Abnormal	Reference
Yeast KOH (seen under the microscope)		Many	None-Rare

Comments: Beneficial flora are normal inhabitants of the intestinal tract and should be found at levels of 3+ or 4 +. Dysbiotic flora, including yeast, should not be found in high levels in the digestive tract. There are many other potentially bad bacteria and yeast not seen here in this sample report. Notice the complete absence of beneficial bacteria (flora) and the overgrowth of the problematic *Pseudomonas aeruginosa* and *Klebsiella,* as well as *Candida,* in this sample patient.

APPENDIX E

IBS Treatment Center Principles and Philosophy

The IBS Treatment Center emphasizes prevention, treatment, and the promotion of optimal health through the use of therapeutic methods that encourage your innate self-healing process. We believe in providing you with the tools and education necessary for you to be able to take personal responsibility for your own health. This includes things as simple as always providing you with a copy of your lab results. We blend centuries-old knowledge of natural, nontoxic therapies with current advances in the understanding of health and medicine.

Our physicians specialize in the treatment of IBS. We see patients with acute and chronic conditions (though we do not serve as an emergency care center) and employ all standard conventional diagnostic tools including physical examination and laboratory tests, and we refer patients to specialists in other areas as necessary and appropriate.

The IBS Treatment Center uses a variety of therapies to promote health and treat disease including diet, therapeutic nutrition, botanical medicine, physical medicine, pharmaceutical medications, lifestyle counseling, and exercise therapy. At the IBS Treatment Center we easily blend modern, state-of-the-art diagnostic and therapeutic procedures and research with ancient and traditional methods. This represents a thoroughly rational, evenhanded balance of tradition, science, and respect for nature, mind, body, and spirit.

Our diagnoses and therapeutics are supported by scientific research drawn from peer-reviewed journals from many disciplines, including conventional medicine, European medicine, clinical nutrition, phytotherapy (botanical medicine), pharmacognosy (drugs), and psychology.

Clinical research into natural therapies has become an increasingly important focus for physicians. Information technology and new concepts in clinical outcomes assessment are particularly well-suited to evaluating the effectiveness of our treatment protocols and are being used in the research branch of our company, the Innate Health Foundation.

The seven principles underlying our medical philosophy are:

1. The Healing Power of Nature: We recognize an inherent healing ability in the body, which is ordered and intelligent. We act to identify and remove obstacles to recovery and to facilitate and augment this healing ability.

2. Identify and Treat the Causes: We seek to identify and remove the underlying causes of illness, rather than to eliminate or merely suppress symptoms.

3. First Do No Harm: We follow three principles to avoid harming our patients: 1) utilize methods and medicinal substances which minimize the risk of harmful side effects; 2) avoid, when possible, the harmful suppression of symptoms; 3) acknowledge and respect the individual's healing process, using the least force necessary to diagnose and treat illness.

4. Doctor as Teacher: We educate the patient and encourage self-responsibility for health. We also acknowledge the therapeutic value inherent in the doctor-patient relationship.

5. Treat the Whole Person: We treat each individual by taking into account physical, mental, emotional, genetic, environmental, and social factors. Since total health also includes spiritual health, we encourage individuals to pursue their personal spiritual path.

6. Prevention: We emphasize disease prevention and the appropriate interventions to prevent illness. We strive to create a healthy world in which humanity may thrive.

7. Wellness: Wellness follows the establishment and maintenance of optimum health and balance. Wellness is a state of being healthy, characterized by positive emotion, thought, and action. Wellness is inherent in everyone, no matter what "dis-eases" are being experienced. If wellness is really recognized and experienced by an individual, it will more quickly heal a given disease than will direct treatment of the disease alone.

BIBLIOGRAPHY

Amadi, B. (2002). Role of food antigen elimination in treating children with persistent diarrhea and malnutrition in Zambia. *Journal of Pediatric Gastroenterology and Nutrition, 34*(Suppl. 1), S54-S56.

Armentia, A., Rodriguez, R., Callejo, A., Martin-Esteban, M., Martin-Santos, J. M., Salcedo, G., Pascual, C., Sanchez-Monge, R., & Pardo, M. (2002). Allergy after ingestion or inhalation of cereals involves similar allergens in different ages. *Clinical and Experimental Allergy, 32*(8), 1216-1222.

Avonts, L., & De Vuyst, L. (2001). Antimicrobial potential of probiotic lactic acid bacteria. *Meded Rijksuniv Gent Fak Landbouwkd Toegep Biol Wet, 66*(3b), 543-550.

Brown, S., Kerrigan, P., & Waterston, T. (2000). A six-year old suffering from constipation. *Practitioner, 244*(1607), 63-68

Carroccio, A., Montalto, G., Custro, N., Notarbartolo, A., Cavataio, F., D'Amico, D., Alabrese, D., & Iacono, G. (2000). Evidence of very delayed clinical reactions to cow's milk in cow's milk-intolerant patients. *Allergy, 55*(6), 574-579.

Cavataio, F., Carroccio, A., & Iacono, G. (2000). Milk-induced reflux in infants less than one year of age. *Journal of Pediatric Gastroenterology and Nutrition, 30*(Suppl.), S36-S44.

Chin, K. C., Tarlow, M. J., & Allfree, A. J. (1983). Allergy to cows' milk presenting as chronic constipation. *British Medical Journal* (Clinical Research Edition), *287*(6405), 1593.

Cremonini, F., Di Caro, S., Santarelli, L., Gabrielli, M., Candelli, M., Nista, E. C., Lupascu, A., Gasbarrini, G., & Gasbarrini, A. (2002) Probiotics in antibiotic-associated diarrhoea. *Digestive and Liver Disease, 34*(Suppl. 2), S78-S80.

Daher, S., Tahan, S., Sole, D., Naspitz, C. K., Da Silva Patricio, F. R., Neto, U. F., & De Morais, M. B. (2001). Cow's milk protein intolerance and chronic constipation in children. *Pediatric Allergy and Immunology, 12*(6), 339-342.

de Boissieu, D., & Dupont, C. (2000). Infant food allergy: Digestive manifestations [Article in French]. *Allergie et Immunologie, 32*(10), 378-380.

Delgado, S., Florez, A. B., & Mayo, B. (2005). Antibiotic susceptibility of *Lactobacillus* and *Bifidobacterium* species from the human gastrointestinal tract. *Current Microbiology, 50*(4), 202-207.

Elmer, G. W. (2001). Probiotics: "Living drugs." *American Journal of Health-System Pharmacy, 58*(12), 1101-1109.

Floch, M. H., & Narayan, R. (2002). Diet in the irritable bowel syndrome. *Journal of Clinical Gastroenterology, 35*(1, Suppl.), S45-S52.

Foster, A. P., Knowles, T. G., Moore, A. H., Cousins, P. D., Day, M. J., & Hall, E. J. (2003). Serum IgE and IgG responses to food antigens in normal and atopic dogs, and dogs with gastrointestinal disease. *Veterinary Immunology and Immunopathology, 93*(3-4), 113-124.

Fox, C. H., & Dang, G. (2004). Probiotics in the prevention and treatment of diarrhea. *Journal of Alternative and Complementary Medicine, 10*(4), 601-603.

Goldin, B. R. (1998). Health benefits of probiotics. *British Journal of Nutrition*, 80(4), S203-S207.

Guarner, F. & Malagelada, J. R. (2003). Gut flora in health and disease. *Lancet, 361*(9356), 512-519.

Heine, R. G., Elsayed, S., Hosking, C. S., Hill, D. J. (2002). Cow's milk allergy in infancy. *Current Opinion in Allergy and Clinical Immunology, 2*(3), 217-225.

Iacono, G., Carroccio, A., Cavataio, F., Montalto, G., Cantarero, M. D., & Notarbartolo, A. (1995). Chronic constipation as a symptom of cow milk allergy. *Journal of Pediatrics, 126*(1), 34-39.

Iacono, G., Cavataio, F., Montalto, G., Florena, A., Tumminello, M., Soresi, M., Notarbartolo, A., & Carroccio, A. (1998). Intolerance of cow's milk and chronic constipation in children. *New England Journal of Medicine, 229*(16), 1100-1104.

Iacono, G., Cavataio, F., Montalto, G., Soresi, M., Notarbartolo, A., & Carroccio, A. (1998). Persistent cow's milk protein intolerance in infants: the changing faces of the same disease. *Clinical and Experimental Allergy, 28*(7), 817-823.

Ishida, Y., Nakamura, F., Kanzato, H., Sawada, D., Hirata, H., Nishimura, A., Kajimoto, O., & Fujiwara, S. (2005). Clinical effects of *Lactobacillus acidophilus* strain L-92 on perennial allergic rhinitis: A double-blind, placebo-controlled study. *Journal of Dairy Science, 88*(2), 527-533.

Jirapinyo, P., Densupsoontorn, N., Thamonsiri, N., & Wongarn, R. (2002). Prevention of antibiotic-associated diarrhea in infants by probiotics. *Journal of the Medical Association of Thailand, 85*(Suppl. 2), S739-S742.

Klein, K. B. (1988). Controlled treatment trials in the irritable bowel syndrome: A critique. *Gastroenterology*, 95, 232-241.

Kokkonen, J., Ruuska, T., Karttunen, T. J., & Niinimaki, A. (2001). Mucosal pathology of the foregut associated with food allergy and recurrent abdominal pains in children. *Acta Paediatrica, 90*(1), 16-21.

Latcham, F., Merino, F., Lang, A., Garvey, J., Thomson, M.A., Walker-Smith, J. A., Davies, S. E., Phillips, A. D., & Murch, S. H. (2003). A consistent pattern of minor immunodeficiency and subtle enteropathy in children with multiple food allergy. *Journal of Pediatrics, 143*(1), 39-47.

Lee, M. C., Lin, L. H., Hung, K. L., & Wu, H. Y. (2001). Oral bacterial therapy promotes recovery from acute diarrhea in children. *Acta Paediatrica Taiwanica, 42*(5), 301-305.

Lembo, A. (2004). Irritable bowel syndrome medications side effects survey. *Journal of Clinical Gastroenterology, 38*(9), 776-781

Magazzu, G., & Scoglio, R. (2002). Gastrointestinal manifestations of cow's milk allergy. *Annals of Allergy, Asthma, & Immunology, 89*(6, Suppl. 1), 65-68.

McGrath, J. (1984). Allergy to cow's milk presenting as chronic constipation. *British Medical Journal* (Clinical Research Edition), *288*(6412), 236.

Moon, A., & Kleinman, R. E. (1995). Allergic gastroenteropathy in children. *Annals of Allergy, Asthma, & Immunology, 74*(1), 5-12.

Mora, W. (2003). Cow's milk protein intolerance and childhood constipation. *American Family Physician, 68*(6), 1016.

Nadasdi, M. (1992). Tolerance of a soy formula by infants and children. *Clinical Therapeutics, 14*(2), 236-241.

Orenstein, S. R., Shalaby, T. M., Di Lorenzo, C., Putnam, P. E., Sigurdsson, L., Mousa, H., & Kocoshis, S. A. (2000). The spectrum of pediatric eosinophilic esophagitis beyond infancy: A clinical series of 30 children. *American Journal of Gastroenterology, 95*(6), 1422-1430.

Pelto, L., Impivaara, O., Salminen, S., Poussa, T., Seppanen, R., & Lilius, E. M. (1999). Milk hypersensitivity in young adults. *European Journal of Clinical Nutrition, 53*(8), 620-624.

Rastall, R. A. (2004). Bacteria in the gut: Friends and foes and how to alter the balance. *Journal of Nutrition, 134*(8, Suppl.), S2022-S2026.

Romanczuk, W., & Samojedny, A. (2003). The assessment of the influence of IgE-mediated food allergy on colonic transit time in children with chronic constipation [Article in Polish]. *Pol Merkuriusz Lek, 15*(87), 226-230.

Saalman, R., Dahlgren, U. I., Fallstrom, S. P., Hanson, L. A., Ahlstedt, S., & Wold, A. E. (2003). Avidity progression of dietary antibodies in healthy and coeliac children. *Clinical and Experimental Immunology, 134*(2), 328-334.

Sabra, A., Bellanti, J. A., Rais, J. M., Castro, H. J., de Inocencio, J. M., & Sabra, S. (2003). IgE and non-IgE food allergy. *Annals of Allergy, Asthma, & Immunology, 90*(6, Suppl. 3), 71-76.

Saggioro, A. (2004). Probiotics in the treatment of irritable bowel syndrome. *Journal of Clinical Gastroenterology, 38*(6, Suppl.), S104-S106.

Salvatore, S., & Vandenplas, Y. (2002). Gastroesophageal reflux and cow milk allergy: Is there a link? *Pediatrics, 110*(5), 972-984.

Shah, N., Lindley, K., & Milla, P. (1999). Cow's milk and chronic constipation in children. *New England Journal of Medicine, 340*(11), 891-892.

Sicherer, S. H. (2003). Clinical aspects of gastrointestinal food allergy in childhood. *Pediatrics, 111*(6, Pt. 3), 1609-1616

Speer, F. (1975). The allergic child. *American Family Physician, 11*(2), 88-94.

Stricker, T., & Braegger, C. P. (2000). Constipation and intolerance to cow's milk. *Journal of Pediatrics Gastroenterology and Nutrition, 30*(2), 224.

Strobel, S, & Hourihane, J. O. (2001). Gastrointestinal allergy: Clinical symptoms and immunological mechanisms. *Pediatric Allergy and Immunology, 12*(Suppl. 14), 43-46.

Taylor, C. J., Hendrickse, R. G., McGaw, J., & Macfarlane, S. B. (1988). Detection of cow's milk protein intolerance by an enzyme-linked immunosorbent assay. *Acta Paediatrica Scandinaica, 77*(1), 49-54.

Vanderhoof, J. A, Perry, D., Hanner, T. L, & Young, R. J. (2001). Allergic constipation: Association with infantile milk allergy. *Clinical Pediatrics, 40*(7), 399-402.

Vanderhoof, J. A., & Young, R. J. (2001). Allergic disorders of the gastrointestinal tract. *Current Opinion in Clinical Nutriton and Metabolic Care, 4*(6), 553-556.

Yimyaem, P., Chongsrisawat, V., Vivatvakin, B., & Wisedopas, N. (2003). Gastrointestinal manifestations of cow's milk protein allergy during the first year of life. *Journal of the Medical Association of Thailand, 86*(2), 116-123.

Zoppi, G. (1996). The most common gastrointestinal problems in pediatric practice [Article in Italian]. *Pediatria Medica e Chirurgica, 18*(2), 131-139.

ABOUT THE AUTHOR

Dr. Stephen Wangen is a state licensed and board certified physician. He received his doctoral degree in naturopathic medicine from the internationally renowned Bastyr University. He practices in Seattle, Washington, and specializes in digestive disorders and food allergies. Due to the tremendous public demand for a solution to the symptoms of irritable bowel syndrome, he founded the Irritable Bowel Syndrome Treatment Center, where he serves as the Chief Medical Officer. In addition to the IBS Treatment Center he has also founded the Center for Food Allergies. His extensive research into the relationship between food allergies and health has led to groundbreaking work on many conditions. He continues to investigate these issues as the Research Director of the Innate Health Foundation, a nonprofit agency dedicated to the advancement of health and health care. His enthusiasm for health care is the result of a lifelong interest in human potential.

INDEX

The Irritable Bowel Syndrome Solution

To order more copies of this book, please use this form or contact us in one of the following ways:

Online: www.ibstreatmentcenter.com
By Mail: 1229 Madison St., Suite 1220, Seattle, WA, 98104
By Phone: IBS Treatment Center, 206-264-1111,
                    Toll free 1-888-546-6283

Name: _____

Address: _____

City: _____

State: _____ Zip: _____

Telephone: (_____) _____

Email address: _____

Price: $14.95 per book. (Add 8.8% tax, or $1.32, for each book shipped within the state of Washington.)

Shipping: U.S. shipping: $4.00 for the first book, $2.00 for each additional book. International shipping: $9.00 for the first book, $5.00 for each additional book.

Number of books requested: _____ x $14.95:   _____

                                    Tax (WA residents only):   _____

                                    Shipping: _____

                                    Total amount: _____

Payment [ ] **Check   Credit:** [ ] Visa or [ ] MC
Please make checks out to Innate Health Services.

Credit Card Number: _____

Exp. Date: _____

Name on Card: _____

Signature: _____